ONE EYE OR TWO?

INSIDER SECRETS TO HELP YOU CHOOSE THE RIGHT LASIK SURGEON

ONE EYE OR TWO?

INSIDER SECRETS TO HELP YOU CHOOSE THE RIGHT LASIK SURGEON

BY

JOHN C. MEYER, MD

and

MARK M. PRUSSIAN

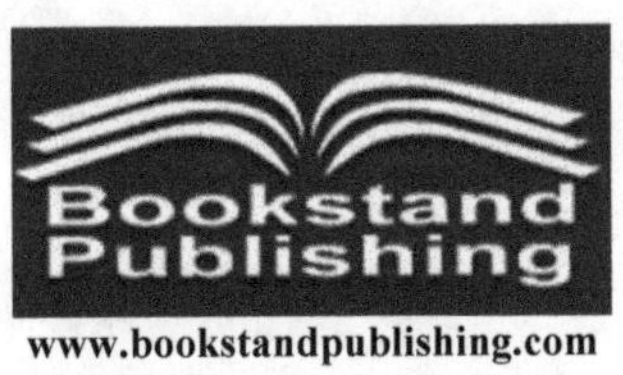

www.bookstandpublishing.com

Published by
Bookstand Publishing
Morgan Hill, CA 95037
4595_2

ISBN 978-1-63498-638-0

Library of Congress Control Number: 2018900186

Printed in the United States of America

DEDICATION AND ACKNOWLEDGEMENTS

To my wife, Donna, for always being my supporter and my partner.

To my children, Emily, Katie, Ellen, and Jack. I am so proud of the young adults each of you have become.

John C. Meyer, MD

To my wife, Betsy, my best friend, confidant, and adviser. I love you more and more each day. Thank you again for always being there for me.

To my daughters, Dana and Dorrie. The times I look forward to most are those I spend with each of you.

To John C. Meyer, MD, and Brennan P. Greene, MD. I could not envision having better business partners and work colleagues. And to Sean F. Murphy, MD, who has since retired, but about whom I share the same feelings.

To the two ophthalmologists from the beginning of my career who offered me a chance in ophthalmic surgery center administration when I was unproven and had only been out of business school a few years. My dedication to create an environment that maximizes the patient-centered experience has its nexus there.

To Taylor Clements, who was instrumental in the layout, design, editing, and production of this book.

To Paul McDonald, who served as an editor of this book.

To work colleagues Caitlin LeMay and Jennifer Miller, who listened and offered advice as I worked on book design and rewrites.

Mark M. Prussian

TABLE OF CONTENTS

Table of Contents

INTRODUCTION

Laser
Assisted
Situ
In
Keratomileusis

LASIK is an acronym that stands for Laser Assisted In Situ Keratomileusis; however, to make it easier to pronounce, the correct Latin term, *in situ*, has been swapped for *situ in*. In situ means "in the place of" and keratomileusis is the shaping of the cornea. So, LASIK literally means laser assistance at the location of the shaping of the cornea.

It is quite natural for prospective LASIK patients to have questions about the success rates of this procedure. A recent study published in the *Journal of Cataract & Refractive Surgery* found that the outcomes for this procedure are now better than ever. The study included 97 LASIK studies and focused on the outcomes of almost 68,000 eyes that had undergone the procedure.

Research from this study found the following:

1. 98.8 percent of patients reported being satisfied with their results.
2. 99.5 percent of eyes attained uncorrected distance visual acuity better than 20/40 after LASIK.
3. 90.9 percent of eyes were within +/- 0.5 diopter (D) of the target refractive outcome.
4. 98.6 percent of eyes were within +/- 1.0 D of the target refractive outcome.

Statistics like these along with anecdotes from actual LASIK patients, coupled with online reviews, show that almost everyone achieves their desired visual result following LASIK.

There are many types of LASIK procedures, each with different benefits, risks, and expected outcomes, and many of them come at different price points. Meeting with an experienced ophthalmologist and a well-trained surgical counselor will allow you to achieve your desired result.

Once you have decided to consider having LASIK, the next step is to find out what is involved in the actual procedure. Very few LASIK patients have access to the detailed explanations and insider information contained in this book. We hope you will read it carefully to help ensure you are making the LASIK decision that is best for you.

Making the decision to have laser eye surgery is one that can help to greatly improve the quality of your life. Your surgeon, along with a talented surgical counselor, can help ensure you are able to enjoy the many benefits that can be provided with laser eye surgery. By understanding precisely what is involved in LASIK, you will be able to determine whether this is the right procedure for your specific vision needs.

So what is the meaning behind *One Eye or Two*? To the ophthalmologist, whether laser vision correction is performed on one eye (monovision) or two eyes (multifocal vision), the technique, skills, training, planning and surgical acumen is the same. From the point of view of the LASIK center operator, however, two eyes cost more to the patient and, therefore, allow more net profit for that LASIK center. As a result, the title *One Eye or Two?* is an acknowledgement that LASIK is a cash-paid, non-insurance-covered procedure yielding higher profits based on greater volume.

CHAPTER 1
THE BASICS OF CORRECTIVE EYE SURGERY

The decision to have corrective eye surgery is certainly an important one and not one that should be taken lightly. You should have all available information in order to determine what is involved so that you can make an informed decision and determine whether this procedure is right for you.

Prior to delving into what is involved in corrective eye surgery, it's vital that you have a solid understanding of the anatomy of the eye and how vision works.

UNDERSTANDING THE ANATOMY OF THE EYE

Given its size, the eye is considered one of the most complex organs in the body. Despite its small size, the human eye contains a number of working parts:

- **Anterior Chamber** – The front section of the interior of the eye. This is where the aqueous humor flows in and out of the eye, providing nourishment.
- **Aqueous Humor** – The clear fluid found in the front of the eye.
- **Blood Vessels** – Arteries and veins that are responsible for transporting blood to and from the eye.
- **Caruncle** – The red part of the corner of the eye. The caruncle contains sweat and sebaceous glands.
- **Choroid** – A thin membrane rich in blood that is located between the sclera and the retina. The choroid is responsible for delivering blood to the retina.

- **Ciliary Body** – This is the part of the eye that is responsible for producing aqueous humor.
- **Cornea** – The clear, dome-shaped front surface of the eye.
- **Iris** – This is the colored part of the eye. It is partially responsible for regulating the amount of light that is allowed to enter the eye.
- **Lens** – Also known as the crystalline lens, this is the transparent structure located inside the eye that is responsible for focusing light rays upon the retina.
- **Lower Eyelid** – The lower skin that covers the front part of the eyeball when the eye is closed.
- **Macula** – The focusing part of the eye. This is what allows us to see fine details.
- **Optic Nerve** – A bundle of nerve fibers that connect the brain to the retina as well as transport light, dark, and color signals to the visual cortex of the brain, which then assembles those signals into images, giving us our vision.
- **Posterior Chamber** – The back portion of the interior of the eye.
- **Pupil** – The opening located in the middle of the iris. Light passes through the pupil to reach the back of the eye.
- **Retina** – A light-sensitive nerve layer lining the back part of the eye. The retina is responsible for sensing light and then creating impulses that are transported through the optic nerve to our brain.
- **Sclera** – This is the white portion of the eyeball that is visible. Attached to the sclera are the muscles that move the eyeball.
- **Stroma** – The thickest layer of the cornea, sandwiched between the epithelium and the inner endothelium.

- **Suspensory Ligament of Lens** – A network of fibers that connect the lens to the ciliary body of the eye to hold it in place.
- **Upper Eyelid** – The top fold of the eye that covers the eyeball when it is closed.
- **Vitreous Body** – A clear substance that has a jelly-like consistency that fills the back of the eye.

THE THREE LAYERS OF THE EYE

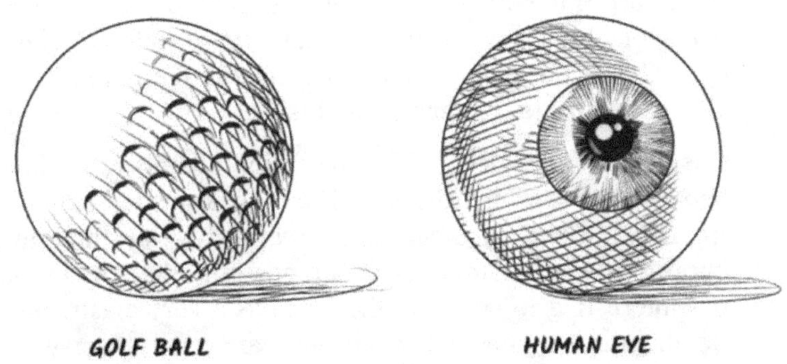

Basically, the eye is shaped similarly to a golf ball with a small bulge located at the front. There are three primary layers to the eye.

<u>Outer Layer</u>

The outer layer is somewhat rough in texture and has a white, tough, opaque membrane known as the sclera. This is the white of the eye. If you look closely at your eye, you might notice a small bulge near the front of the eye. This thin, clear, dome-shaped tissue is the cornea of the eye.

<u>Middle Layer</u>

The middle layer of the eye is the choroid. At the front of the choroid is the iris, which is the colored part of the eye. The pupil is located in the center of the iris.

Inner Layer

The inner layer of the eye is the retina, which consists of two layers. Those layers are the sensory retina, which contains nerve cells that are responsible for processing visual information and transmitting to the brain, and the retinal pigment epithelium or RPE, which is located between the eyewall and the sensory retina.

SECTIONS OF THE EYE

The interior of the eye is divided into three sections known as chambers. These chambers include the following components:

- **Anterior Chamber** – The anterior chamber is located in the front part of the eye between the iris and the cornea. The iris is responsible for controlling the amount of light entering the eye. This is done by opening and closing the pupil. The iris also uses muscles to change pupil size.
- **Posterior Chamber** – The posterior chamber is situated between the lens and the iris. The lens is located behind the iris and is typically clear. Light makes its way through the pupil to the lens. Small tissue strands hold the lens in place. It's interesting to note that the lens has a very elastic nature. Small muscles attached to the lens are used to change the shape of the lens, which make it possible for the eye to focus on objects at different distances. This is known as accommodation.
- **Vitreous Chamber** – Between the back of the eye and the lens is the vitreous chamber. The back two-thirds of this chamber is lined with special cells. These incredibly sensitive nerve cells are responsible for converting light into nerve impulses. It is the nerve fibers located in the retina that come together to form the optic nerve, which is connected to the brain. Nerve impulses are transported through this nerve to the brain. Near the center of the retina, at the back of the eye, is the macula, which is responsible for giving us sharp, detailed vision. The remainder of the retina is responsible for delivering side or peripheral vision, which makes it possible for us to see shapes, although not fine details. Blood vessels,

including the retinal artery and vein, make their way along the optic nerve before exiting the back of the eye.

Much of the inside of the eye is filled with fluid. The clear, watery fluid that fills the anterior and posterior chambers is known as aqueous humor, whereas a thick, jelly-like fluid known as vitreous humor fills the vitreous chamber. These two different types of fluids actually press against the interior of the eyeball to give it proper shape.

HOW THE EYE WORKS

The human eye works much like a camera. Light passes through the cornea and the pupil located at the front of the eye. From there, the lens focuses light onto the retina, situated at the back of the eye. The cornea and the lens bend the light so it can pass through the thick vitreous gel located in the posterior chamber and then projects onto the retina. From there, the retina converts light into electrical impulses. These electrical impulses are transported by the optic nerve to the brain. Finally, the brain converts the electric pulses into the images that we see. While it certainly sounds like a complicated process, and it is, it happens extremely quickly.

To put it in the perspective of a camera, the cornea acts somewhat like the lens of a camera by primarily focusing light. The eye's iris works similarly to a camera diaphragm by controlling the amount of light that reaches the back of the eye. This is done by adjusting the size of the pupil automatically, like the aperture of a camera. The crystalline lens of the eye, which is situated directly behind the pupil, is responsible for further focusing light.

A process known as accommodation works to assist the eye in focusing on both near and approaching objects automatically, sort of like an autofocus camera lens. In many ways, the retina works similar to the electronic image sensor on a digital camera. It converts optical images into electronic signals. These signals are then transmitted by the optic nerve to the visual cortex, which is the part of the brain that is responsible for controlling our sense of light.

HOW CORRECTIVE EYE SURGERY HAS EVOLVED

Now that we have a good idea of the anatomy of the eye and how the eye functions, it's a good idea to explore how corrective eye surgery has evolved over the years. Historically speaking, attempts to correct vision refractive problems date back several centuries.

The History of Ophthalmology

Laser vision correction surgery has had a long history. For centuries, humans have sought ways to correct their vision. The first eyeglasses made their appearance in Italy during the 13th century. Many years later, in 1888, contact lenses were developed in Switzerland. Despite these revolutionary innovations, physicians were still looking for a more permanent solution to correct vision problems.

Many people might be surprised to discover that ophthalmology was somewhat advanced in ancient Egypt as early as 1600 B.C., at least in comparison to other medical specializations at the time. While a number of vision conditions had already been recognized, there were few treatment options available – and those that *were* available were hardly sophisticated. Some even involved the use of lizard blood.

During the second century A.D., Galen, a prominent Greek physician, penned a number of texts on the subject of ophthalmology. According to his theories, light rays made their way from the brain through the optic nerve to the retina, lens, and cornea. He also speculated that these same rays could then return along the same path, thus producing vision.

Hermann von Helmholtz, a Viennese scientist, invented the ophthalmoscope in 1854. As a result, it became possible to obtain direct visualization of the eye's interior. Use of the new instrument proved to be challenging and time-consuming. As a result, few general surgeons used it. A few patient physicians had the fortitude to stick with it, which ultimately led to the creation of ophthalmology as a specialty.

The current device most people are familiar with to check the need for vision correction, the phoropter, was invented in 1909. It went through several rapid improvements and has remained, mostly unchanged for the past 100 years. This is the instrument the doctor or technician will use to determine your prescription. You may be most familiar with the phoropter as this is the instrument with which you hear the phrases "Better A or better B or about the same?" or "Better one or better two or about the same?"

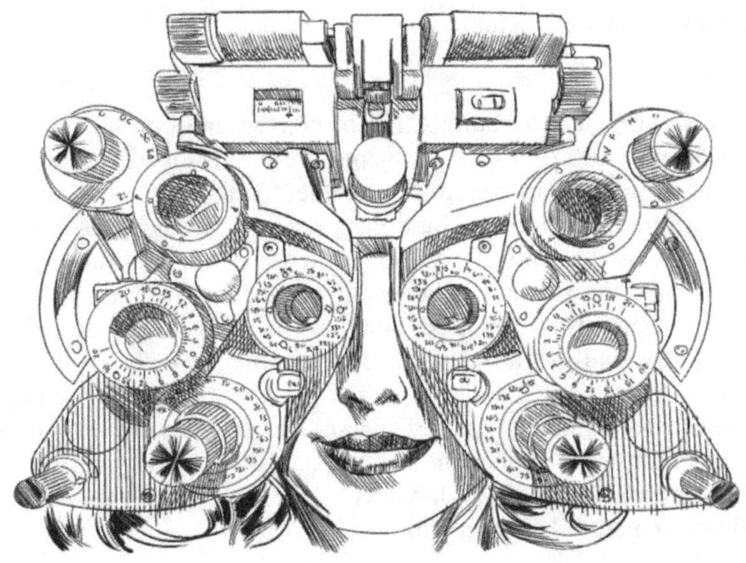

PHOROPTER

As ophthalmology became its own specialty, research into the field continued. A Dutch professor, Frans Cornelius Donders, was among the first to use the ophthalmoscope to study the human eye.

His work in this emerging new field led other physicians to gain interest in ophthalmology as well.

Early Glasses and Contacts

Glass lenses, dating back to 300 BC, were originally used as magnifiers and for lighting fires. It was not until 1280 in Florence, Italy, that eyeglasses were first used for the purpose of aiding or correcting vision. The lenses were convex and worn by physicist Salvino degli Armati, who had injured his own eyes as a result of light refraction experiments.

During the early 14th century, concave lenses were first used for the purposes of correcting nearsightedness. Pope Leo X has been depicted as wearing concave lens glasses. At the time, early eyeglasses were constructed of polished quartz; however, by the 16th century, glassmaking developments made it possible to mass produce eyeglasses that were actually made from glass.

Bifocals

Bifocals, which are a combination of convex and concave lenses to correct both types of vision problems, were developed around 1760. This new innovation made it possible to achieve clear distance viewing through a top lens and ease reading through a lower lens. Using two distinct optical powers, the lenses are sometimes referred to as Benjamin Franklin glasses in recognition of the man who invented them. It is reported that Franklin developed the glasses because he had begun experiencing problems with seeing at a distance as well as up close. After growing weary of switching between two different types of glasses, he found a way to fit both into a single frame. Later, the trifocal lenses were invented by John Isaac Hawkins in 1824. Hawkins coined the term bifocals and credited Benjamin Franklin with their invention.

Originally, bifocals were designed in such a way that the convex lenses for close viewing were situated in the lower half while the convex lenses were located in the upper half of the frame. Two separate lenses were usually cut in half and then pieced together in the rim of the frame. As a result, bifocals tended to be quite fragile. It was not until the early 20th century that this changed. Today, these glasses, called multifocal glasses, are most commonly prescribed for people with presbyopia, or farsightedness, who also require a myopia, or nearsightedness, correction or who have an astigmatism.

Early Ophthalmology

The eye has remained the subject of consideration and research since the early days of history.

> *"The eye is like a mirror, and the visible object is like the thing reflected in the mirror." – Avicenna, 11th century Persian philosopher*

A number of ancient philosophers and physicians believed in the concept of an active eye. In the fourth century B.C., Plato wrote that light actually emanated from the eye. A disciple of Aristotle, Theophrastus, theorized that the eye had fire within it, departing from the beliefs of his teacher. Aristotle had been among the first to reject the idea that seeing takes place by something that is issued *from* the eye. In fact, Aristotle strongly advocated for the idea that the eye *received* rays rather than issued them.

During the second century A.D., one of the most prominent ancient physicians, Galen, offered multiple theories related to the eye and vision. It was his thoughts on vision that continued to define many ideas regarding the physiology and anatomy of the eye up until the 17th century. Galen described the cornea, retina, uvea, iris, eyelids, and tear ducts, along with two fluids that he named the vitreous and aqueous humors. In his work, he also noted binocular vision and was particularly interested in the idea of the crystalline lens. According to Galen, "The crystalline lens is the principal instrument of vision, a fact clearly proved by what physicians call cataracts, which lie between the crystalline humor and the cornea and interfere with vision until they are couched."

Vision continued to be a subject of special interest to Islamic scholars between the 9th and 14th centuries. During that time, multiple treatises on the subject of ophthalmology appeared. Many scholars of the time were heavily influenced by Galen, including al-Kindi. Works at the time paid special attention to the retina.

The details of the eye were actively debated by Islamic physicians. During the 10th century, al-Razi, a Baghdad clinician, noted the contraction and dilation of the pupil. A century later, the ability of the eye to be injured by strong light was noted by al-Haythan. By this time, it had come to be accepted that the eye was affected by light rather than light being affected by the eye.

During the 11th and 12th centuries, the rich body of work related to ophthalmology was translated into Latin from Arabic. As European medical researchers began to ponder their own theories regarding the eye and how it worked, Nicolaus, a Persian mathematician, wrote in the late 12th century that, "The optic nerve, which descends from the brain to the eyes, passes through the center of the eye as far as the crystalline humor, through it comes the visible spirit, and as it emerges through the uveal tonic and the cornea, it is mingled with clean air and transports its rays to the body, and thus sight is brought about."

Divided Theories During the Renaissance

Anatomists working during the Renaissance learned a tremendous amount about the eye's anatomy.

At the time, theories regarding vision were primarily divided into two categories. One group believed in the concept of extramission, meaning that something leaves the eyes when we see something. Another group argued the intromission theory, meaning that vision takes place by something entering the eyes.

During the fifth century BCE, the Greek philosopher Empedocles contended that vision took place when light was issued from the eyes, referring to the theory of extramission. Plato had varyingly supported both theories in the following century. Aristotle also tended to swing back and forth in favor of intromission versus extramission. Even though there had been a growing tendency favoring the concept of intromission, the idea of something leaving the eyes when vision occurred did not completely disappear. Leonardo da Vinci advocated for the theory of extramission in the 1480s. At the time, many adults and children had a particular fear of what was known as the evil eye, seeming to reinforce the idea that something leaves the eye as part of the vision process.

A decade later, da Vinci reversed his position. He wrote, "The eye, the instrument of vision, is hidden in the cavity above, and in that below is the humor which nourishes the roots of the teeth." Even he had a fascination with the effect of light on the eye and spent some time examining the pupil.

During the 16th century, theories regarding sight varied somewhat. For instance, Italian philosopher and physician Alessandro Achillini, became one of the first people to challenge the concept that the crystalline lens was the main source of sight. Vesalius, a Flemish anatomist, continued to advocate for the concept that the crystalline lens was responsible for sight but argued that the optic nerves were not hollow.

Later, anatomists began examining the crystalline humor more closely, noticing that it was more oblong in shape rather than round and located more toward the front of the eye. Felix Platter, a Swiss physician, argued in 1583 that the optic nerve should be considered the primary vision organ.

The first theory of retinal image was not advanced until 1604, when German mathematician and astronomer Johannes Kepler promoted the idea, stating, "vision occurs through a picture of the visible things on the white, concave surface of the retina."

Ophthalmology Becomes a Specialty in Its Own Right

Although the first cataract surgery was performed more than 2,000 years ago in India by a surgeon named Susruta, it was not until the mid-19th century in Europe that ophthalmology became recognized as an established medical specialty. At that time, a number of scientific advances in the vision field had been made, as researchers were developing an understanding of refractive errors as well as how to correct those errors.

The continued research and expansion of the ophthalmology field led to the founding of what is now known as the American Academy of Ophthalmology in 1864. The organization was the first of its kind in the United States. Ophthalmology became the first medical branch to develop specialty board exams in 1917. Ophthalmology was recognized as the first medical specialty when it separated from otolaryngology (ear, nose, and throat) at the beginning of the 20th century.

The Development of Corrective Eye Surgery

It was also around the end of the 19th century that the first research was published regarding how vision could be improved other than just wearing glasses. It was around this time that researchers began looking at what could be done to reshape the cornea to improve visual acuity.

In 1948, polish missionary and ophthalmologist, Father Waclaw Szuniewicz pioneered refractive surgery of the cornea when he discovered how to change corneal curvature. After traveling to the

United States, he continued experimental work on his surgical method at Yale University.

HISTORY OF LASIK EYE SURGERY

Some of the earliest laser eye surgeries were performed in Colombia by Dr. Jose Barraquer in the 19th century. A medical field pioneer, Barraquer had a specific interest in experimenting with corneal tissue. It was his belief that it was possible to help patients see clearly by making certain adjustments to the cornea. Far ahead of his time, Barraquer first performed experiments to make the transition from previously accepted barbaric customs to techniques that were more modern and safer. Barraquer was the first to introduce the microkeratome. This tool began the transition from making manual incisions with a scalpel to mechanized cuts with a stabilized blade (still used in low-priced LASIK). The most modern technology today uses a sophisticated laser that takes thousands of measurements prior to creating the flap for LASIK, rather than a manual or stabilized blade (often called a keratome).

Barraquer's procedure was accomplished using three steps. First, the cornea would be cut open. Next, a disk would be removed using the microkeratome. It would then be reshaped and re-attached using a cryo lathe. At the time, the technique represented a tremendous step forward, but it was still not as precise as was needed. Additionally, rehabilitation could be lengthy.

Laser Vision Enters the Scene

The history of laser vision surgery dates back to the development and testing of lasers, specifically the excimer laser. The word laser is actually an acronym that stands for "light amplification by stimulated emission of radiation." The term excimer comes from "excited dimer," an extremely small particle. When the particle breaks down, it creates energy and ultraviolet light.

There were a number of failed experiments up until about 1974, when radial keratotomy (RK) was developed. RK is the practice of making actual incisions on the surface of the cornea in a sort of spoke-like design. The result of this radial incision was a central flattening of the cornea. Interestingly, this procedure was the result of an accidental discovery by a Soviet ophthalmologist, Svyatoslav Fyodorov, who observed that a change in refraction occurred in a patient after the patient experienced eye trauma as a result of broken glasses. The lacerations on his patient's eyes occurred in a radial design, and after the lacerations were healed, the patient reported a significant reduction in his previous myopia. It was sometime during the late 1970s the Soviet military made the decision to actually force Russian soldiers to have the procedure because it was less expensive for the military as well as less hassle than getting glasses for soldiers. It became sort of an assembly line approach.

After learning of the research being done in the Soviet Union, Dr. Leo Bores from Detroit, Michigan, made the trip to visit Dr. Fyodorov many times at his clinic before he began performing the procedure in the United States beginning in 1978.

What Is the Excimer Laser?

IBM's development of the excimer laser proved to be a crucial development that eventually made laser eye surgery possible. Excimer lasers take their name from the terms "excited" and "dimers." Because these lasers are cool lasers, they do not heat up adjacent surfaces or the surrounding air. Rather, they emit an incredibly focused beam of ultraviolet light. The upper surface that comes into contact with it absorbs this light. For most organic materials, the vast amount of ultraviolet light is simply too much to absorb. As a result, the molecular bonds of the material simply break down.

How a Computer Company Helped Us All See Better

The next big development that occurred in the field of laser correction surgery took place between 1970 and 1980. It was actually due to some leftover turkey dinner the day after Thanksgiving Day in 1981 that the lives of literally millions of people would be changed forever. Three IBM researchers had been exploring new ways in which the excimer laser, which their chemistry and laser physics group had recently acquired, could be used. This is the same laser that forms the basis of what we use for LASIK today.

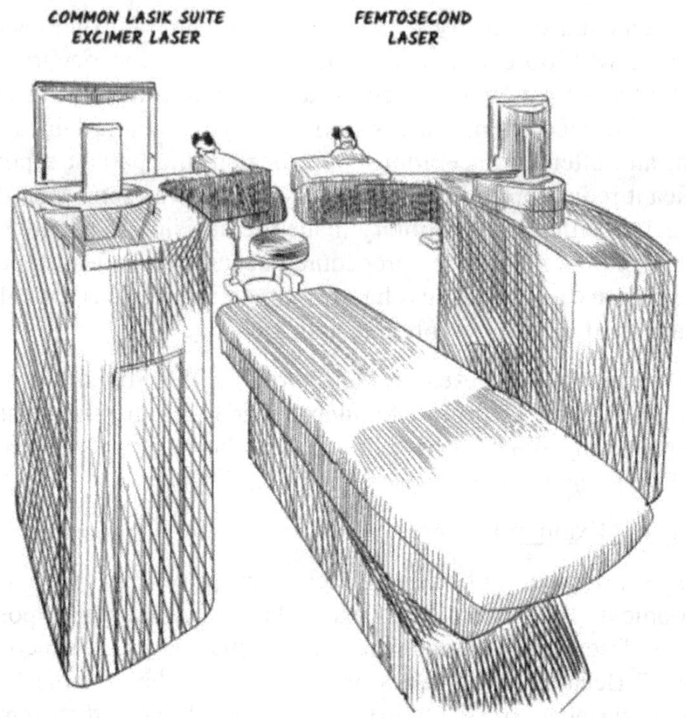

Samuel Blum, Rangaswamy Srinivasan, and James J. Wynne were all working at the Thomas J. Watson Research Center in Yorktown, New York. Wynne, a physicist, managed the group at IBM, Blum was a materials science expert, and Srinivasan was a photo chemist with almost two dozen US patents to his name.

The excimer laser became commercially available in 1979. After the group acquired one of the lasers, it was installed in Peter Sorokin's lab, the first such laser in use at IBM. Freely encouraged to use the laser, the group began to toss around different options. However, one thing they were afraid to do was actually shine it on their own skin. That concern eventually led to discussions of other types of tissue that could be used for experimenting with the laser. Initially, they did experiment on their own fingernails, discovering that the laser had the ability to produce incredibly precise patterns etched in keratin, the tough protein that comprises fingernails. The experiment came to a halt when the researchers balked at the idea of actually removing their fingernails for further experimentation.

The excimer laser uses reaction gases, including fluorine and chlorine, mixed with various inert gases, such as krypton, argon, and xenon. When the gases are electrically excited, the mixture produces energetic pulses of ultraviolet light. That light has the capability of producing incredibly precise, although extremely small, changes to irradiated materials.

According to Wynne, the group wondered if the excimer laser would be effective on human or animal tissues. The breakthrough really occurred when the group discussion turned to the type of tissue that could be used. It was Srinivasan who brought his Thanksgiving turkey leftovers to the lab the day after Thanksgiving to give it a trial run. The group immediately knew they had discovered a new form of surgery. By directing the ultraviolet light from the excimer laser, the scientists were able to achieve an extremely clean incision without damaging surrounding tissue.

Using a succession of short laser pulses, they were able to remove tissue. They discovered that the laser had the remarkable ability to cut extremely precise yet smooth grooves. A combination of fluorine and argon gases by the excimer eye surgery laser to produce an invisible ultraviolet light beam. By using a series of lenses and mirrors, it's possible to focus the laser light to produce a smooth, even beam. Very little heat is produced by this laser, which means there is little heat damage to nearby tissues.

After the group signed an invention disclosure in 1981 and filed a patent application the following year, they finally worked up enough courage to use the laser on their own skin. Wynne held up his pinky finger and shone the laser directly on it. With every pulse of the laser, a thin layer of his tissue was removed, yet he reported feeling no sense of pain or heat. The only sensation he felt was some pressure. From that point, Wynne began collaborating with dermatologists and went on to publish multiple papers about the uses of the excimer laser.

After learning of the research being performed at IBM using the excimer laser, American ophthalmologist Dr. Stephen Trokel traveled to the Watson Research Center in 1983 to work with the group.

Trokel began to collaborate with experts and experiment with the excimer laser. Among those collaborations was an experiment in which they irradiated the cornea of a cow eye using the excimer laser. Once again, they were able to produce clean incisions without any damage to adjacent tissues. Trokel was the first person to use the laser on corneal tissue at Columbia University in New York. He was impressed with the results produced by the laser as well as its possibilities.

What followed was years of experimentation and clinical trials. It was not until 1995 that the Food and Drug Administration finally granted approval for the first excimer laser-based refractive surgery system.

Trokel, Srinivasen, and researcher Bodil Braren continued their experiments and later wrote a paper that would introduce the concept of using the excimer laser to sculpt or reshape the cornea for the purpose of correcting refractive vision errors. This paper went on to be published in an ophthalmology journal in late 1983. It was that paper that inspired ophthalmologists from around the world to begin using the excimer laser for correcting astigmatism, myopia, and hyperopia.

In 1985, Dr. Theo Seiler performed the first excimer laser patient procedure in Germany. During the procedure, he attempted to create corneal incisions in a manner similar to RK. Later, it was found that the excimer laser was more effective at removing central tissue on the cornea to create a flattening effect. The removal of tissue by a laser is known as photoablation. Molecular bonds break down, causing tissue to literally disintegrate. The process of applying laser photoablation directly to the corneal central surface eventually became known as photorefractive keratotomy (PRK). In 1987, a blind patient became the first individual to undergo the procedure at Columbia University. The following year, Dr. Marguerite McDonald performed the first PRK procedure on a non-blind patient at Louisiana State University.

Although the procedure was proven to be effective, PRK was somewhat slow to gain popularity. It was not until laser in situ keratomileusis (LASIK) was introduced and became routine that the popularity of laser eye vision surgery began to soar. With LASIK, patients were able to enjoy the benefits of having their vision corrected quickly while experiencing very little, if any, pain.

In 1995, the first laser received approval by the FDA for general use. Since that time, numerous other lasers have received approval from the FDA. Today, older lasers are usually referred to in the industry as either first-generation or second-generation lasers. These lasers typically utilize broad-beam laser technology. More modern lasers use scanning spot technology. As a result, they are able to offer an array of treatments. Among the benefits of these lasers is their ability to produce a larger optical zone and smoother surface. This helps to reduce nighttime halos and glares.

James Wynne has since received numerous Outstanding Innovation Awards and was inducted into the National Inventors Hall of Fame, along with Samuel Blum and Rangaswamy Srinivasan.

INTRODUCING THE POSSIBILITIES TO THE WORLD

The team knew they would need to demonstrate what they had discovered. They elected to use a highly magnified electron micrographic image of one strand of human hair that the laser had etched. Eventually, that image made its way into publications around the world.

Moving forward, the trio had a number of discussions regarding the best way to utilize the new clean excision they had discovered in a surgical format. For instance, would it be used for dentistry, brain surgery, dermatology, or something else?

Research at the time was ongoing for an alternative for the surgical procedure currently in use for correcting nearsightedness. The use of a scalpel had a number of drawbacks, including the fact that it was not at all precise and could result in permanent weakening of the cornea.

Over the course of the next ten years, the ophthalmology community continued to work diligently at perfecting both the equipment and the techniques used in laser eye surgery.

PRK became the first type of corrective eye surgery to utilize a laser instead of a blade for the removal of corneal tissue. While the excimer laser had been developed in the early 1970s and later modified for the use of ophthalmologic surgery in the early 1980s, the FDA did not approve it for use in PRK surgery until 1995.

Originally, PRK was used for treating myopia by removing a small amount of the cornea. Later, technological refinements made it possible for patients with astigmatism and farsightedness to be treated using this procedure. There is no need to create a flap in PRK. Instead, the surgeon applies the laser directly to the corneal surface. Consequently, the recovery period using this procedure is longer and more uncomfortable.

Since the advent of LASIK, a number of other innovations in the field of vision correction surgery have taken place. Dr. Tibo Juhasz, a biomedical engineer, began experimenting with the femtosecond laser in 1997. It was later approved for use in the United States for bladeless LASIK, gaining approval from the FDA in 2001. This femtosecond laser has commonly replaced the manual keratome in all but the lowest-priced LASIK centers.

As a result of the minimal amount of pain and rapid healing cycle it offers, LASIK is now the most popular vision correction surgery in the world (American Refractive Surgery Council). Millions of people have undergone the procedure, with a vast majority enjoying excellent vision along with the ability to go about their daily activities without the need to rely on contact lenses or glasses.

WHAT HAPPENS DURING LASIK?

Now, that we have talked about how LASIK evolved and some basic background regarding what is involved, let's take a closer look at the two-step process called LASIK.

Step One: Use of the Femtosecond Laser

Once you've made the decision to have LASIK, the day of surgery finally arrives. You'll be taken into an exam room where the surgeon and LASIK team will make sure that all of your questions have been answered and that you are comfortable. In that exam room, you will meet with the surgeon to verify your measurements and desired outcome while the technician instills eye drops. You will have a final opportunity to ask the surgeon any questions you may have.

Once you are in the LASIK suite, the team will have you lie on your back in a reclining chair and position you under the laser system. The LASIK team, which consists of the surgeon and two or three other staff members, will verify the measurements placed into the laser system's computer. You should expect your surgeon to be speaking with you and the LASIK team during the entire procedure to keep you updated on your progress. An instrument, referred to as a lid speculum, will keep your eyelids open during the procedure.

The femtosecond laser is used to create the flap. After this, the reclining chair will gently move you about two feet so that you are positioned under the excimer laser.

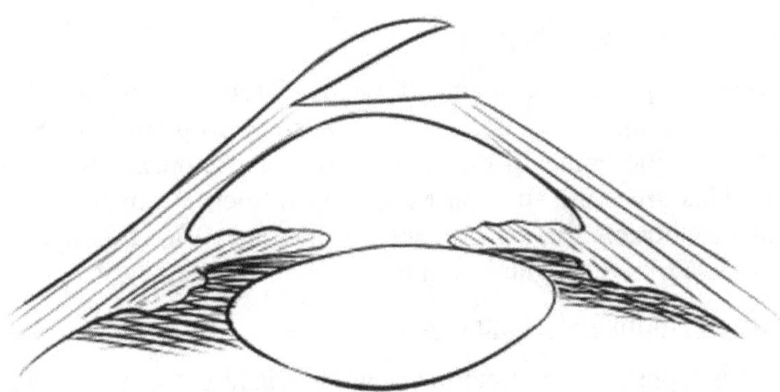

Step Two: Use of the Excimer Laser

After the creation of the flap, it is folded back to reveal the stroma or underlying cornea. This allows the surgeon to use the excimer laser to remove the appropriate amount of corneal tissue. The laser utilizes a cool ultraviolet light beam to remove microscopic amounts of tissue to reshape the cornea.

Once the surgeon has put the flap back into place and smoothed the cornea, he or she will then apply a special solution to help the flap refloat for proper placement. The cornea begins sealing itself within just a few minutes while you then rest in the reclining chair for a few minutes. Then anti-inflammatory and antibiotic drops are applied to your eyes. After this is done, the reclining chair is gently moved about two feet so that it is once again underneath the femtosecond laser and treatment of your second eye can begin.

DIFFERENCES IN LASER TREATMENTS

There are several ways the cornea can be reshaped during refractive surgery:

Traditional Standard Treatment

In the traditional approach, the cornea is reshaped using approximately the same measurements for contacts or glasses. This approach is used to treat nearsightedness, farsightedness, and astigmatism.

Wavefront Guided Treatment

In wavefront guided treatment, the same issues are treated as with the traditional approach along with higher-order aberrations. Several thousand unique points of the patient's vision are measured to create a map. This gives the surgeon the ability to measure distortions that cannot be corrected using contacts or glasses. With this approach, it's possible to reduce glares and halos while sharpening vision.

Wavefront Optimized Treatment

With this approach, a treatment pattern is created that helps to maintain the round, natural curve of the eye while producing crisp, sharp vision. This treatment approach also helps to lessen nighttime halos and glares following the surgery. Wavefront optimized treatment uses more laser pulses in the periphery of the cornea to minimize visual distortion due to the curved shape of the cornea.

Topography Guided Treatment

With this approach, an advanced corneal topographer device is used to map 22,000 unique elevations of the cornea, allowing for a superbly customized LASIK treatment plan.

The Advantages of LASIK over PRK

As is the case with PRK, LASIK presents its own advantages and disadvantages. This is largely because LASIK involves a second procedure, the creation of a flap, which is known as keratectomy. Over the years, as the microkeratome evolved into the femtosecond laser, LASIK has become the preferred procedure for laser vision correction. Femtosecond lasers, such as the Alcon FS200, which creates thousands of data points before the procedure begins, have caused near-perfect vision correction.

Different Types of LASIK AND PRK

In deciding whether vision correction surgery is right for your needs, you may be interested in learning about the different variations of both LASIK and PRK.

Other Forms of LASIK

You may hear terms like LASEK, Epi-LASIK, Wavefront LASIK, or similar procedures. These are all variations of LASIK, either using brand names of laser manufacturers or using tweaks of surgical procedures, which have become branded names by the ophthalmologist who created the tweak. The best procedure to improve your vision is going to happen when you meet with your LASIK surgeon at each visit so that together you and your surgeon can agree on the procedure that's right for you.

MISPERCEPTIONS ABOUT LASIK

The most common misperception is that there will be pain and bleeding. This is not true. A well-known physician who hosts his own medical TV show produced a trailer for an episode on LASIK. The trailer, viewed over two million times, falsely showed bleeding eyelids as a hook to get viewers. LASIK, and all other refractive procedures, are actually bloodless.

Another misperception is that people think it will take a long period of time for their vision to stabilize, and it really doesn't. It's often stabilized in 45–90 minutes after the procedure.

Another misperception that people have is that they will be put to sleep during the procedure. Actually, the LASIK surgeon will give you a small dose of medication to make you forget what happened during the procedure.

Are you ready to learn more about LASIK and find out whether you might be a good candidate for LASIK? If so, keep reading. In the next chapter, we are going to debunk some LASIK myths; discuss risk factors; determine who might be a good candidate for LASIK; and discuss the types of vision errors that can be corrected with LASIK, what to expect from your initial consultation, possible side effects, and expected results.

CHAPTER 2

MAKING THE DECISION TO HAVE LASIK

The decision to have LASIK is not a decision that should be taken lightly. As with any medical procedure, having all of the facts can help you make an informed decision regarding whether this is the best procedure for your particular situation.

ARE YOU A GOOD CANDIDATE FOR LASIK?

It should be understood that while LASIK can help many people eliminate the need to wear glasses or use contacts, it is not for everyone. Often ophthalmologists can restore vision to a point where the patient is really satisfied, regardless of the common—but not always useful—measure of being able to read 20/20 on the Snellen visual acuity chart. These patients are often referred to as "20/Happy." Therefore, it's important to determine whether you are a good candidate for LASIK and to make sure you, and your surgeon, agree to vision achievement goals.

MARKET-TO-METHOD DISPARITY

Before we delve into whether you are personally a good candidate for LASIK, it's important to first discuss what is known as market-to-method disparity and understanding 20/20 vision. Most people think that when it comes to vision, 20/20 is the goal. There's even a cliché about hindsight being 20/20. There is a better, healthier way to look at it.

IS 20/20 VISION GOOD? ®

What exactly is 20/20, and why do so many people think that when it comes to great vision, 20/20 is guiding standard? 20/20 vision refers to how well you can see a line that has been marked at 20 feet away.

This is a visual acuity chart, which was actually developed by Hermann Snellen, a Dutch eye doctor, back in the 1860s. Today, there are numerous variations of this eye chart, but almost all of them display 11 rows of capital letters. One letter is featured on the top row. This is usually a big letter E, but you could use any letter. The letters become progressively smaller moving down the rows. The visual acuity chart is used by eye doctors to measure how well patients are able to see in the distance. An eye doctor will usually ask you to locate the smallest line of letters you are able to see clearly and read those letters.

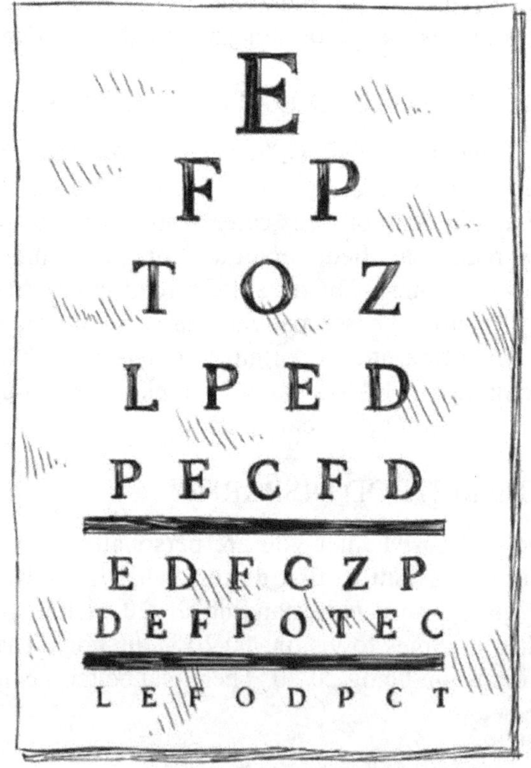

SNELLEN VISUAL ACUITY EYE CHART

Eye charts in the United States are designed for placement on a wall that is located 20 feet from the patient. The problem is that the exam rooms (often called exam lanes) in most eye doctor offices are not 20 feet in length. You might see an eye chart hanging on a wall behind a chair or the doctor might even use mirrors to simulate a distance of 20 feet.

While 20/20 vision is considered to be normal vision, in its simplest form, this just gives us a standard way to measure vision. This means you are able to comfortably read text located at 20 feet away from you. Let's use the big letter E at the top of a standard 20/200 eye chart as an example. If you are only able to read this letter from 20 feet away, you would be considered to have 20/200 vision. This means you are able to read a letter from 20 feet away that people who are considered to have normal vision are able to read at a distance of 200 feet.

The line for 20/20 vision is typically located fourth from the bottom. The lines for 20/15, 20/10, and 20/5 vision are located below that line. Most people do not have 20/10 visual acuity, so you shouldn't feel bad if your vision is not 20/10. In order to obtain a driver's license in the US, you will usually need to have at least 20/40 vision.

Of course, there are other types of eye charts that are sometimes used. The Snellen visual acuity chart is just one commonly used eye chart. Another is the Tumbling E eye chart. This eye chart is sometimes used in situations in which the Snellen eye chart is not appropriate. For instance, a young child obviously would not be able to use the Snellen chart because he or she may not know the alphabet yet. Individuals who have a handicap or who are illiterate might also benefit more from the Tumbling E chart than the Snellen chart. The Tumbling E chart includes the same scale as is used on the Snellen chart, but every letter on the chart is the letter E. The only difference is that they are situated in different spatial orientations. The patient would be asked to use their hands to indicate the direction the E is pointing.

Another eye chart sometimes used is the Jaeger Eye chart. This eye chart features short blocks of text that are printed in various sizes. Originally developed in 1867, the Jaeger eye chart has undergone a number of modifications over the years. Today, this chart is produced by a number of manufacturers who utilize their own modifications.

Regardless of the type of chart that is used, it's important to understand that all eye charts have some limitations. The biggest problem is that an eye chart is designed to measure only visual acuity. An eye chart can be helpful for determining whether you might need contact lenses or eyeglasses to improve your distance vision. Additionally, the Department of Motor Vehicles finds eye charts helpful for determining whether you need to wear corrective lenses while driving or whether you should even be prohibited from driving if you are legally blind.

The real issue is that eye charts are not able to measure depth perception, peripheral vision, the ability to perceive contrast, or color perception. All of these elements are important to your vision. Furthermore, an eye chart cannot measure your eye health, such as whether you have glaucoma, your eye fluid pressure, the health of your retina or macula, or whether you might suffer from dry eyes. Therefore, it should be understood that while an eye chart can be important, it is just one part of a comprehensive eye exam. Patients with 20/20 vision might not have healthy eyes or may not be satisfied with their vision; 20/20 is one of many measures of eye health and vision rather than the end goal.

DOES 20/20 VISION MATTER?

When people hear 20/20 or better, such as 20/15 or 20/10, they think it is both good vision and good overall eye health. The Snellen visual acuity chart, does not, in any manner, measure your total eye health.

Eye charts measure only visual acuity, which is just one component of good vision. They cannot determine if your eyes are working overtime (needing to focus more than normal, which can lead to headaches and eye strain) or if your eyes are working properly as a team (sometimes called stereovision, for clear, comfortable binocular vision and accurate depth perception). As previously mentioned, eye charts also cannot detect serious eye problems such as glaucoma or early diabetic retinopathy that could lead to serious vision impairment and even blindness. Only a comprehensive eye exam performed by a licensed optometrist or ophthalmologist can determine if your eyes are healthy and you are seeing as clearly and comfortably as possible.

Everyone reading this has heard the term 20/20. But what does it mean? Is 20/20 vision ideal? Do you really want 20/20 vision? Specifically, 20/20 simply means you are able to read a certain line on the Snellen eye chart from 20 feet away. While this is an accurate way to test visual acuity, the Snellen eye chart does not test for other visual aspects of your eye health, such as peripheral vision, depth perception, color perception, or eye coordination.

With age, the ability to have "perfect" vision often declines. Generally, a 50-year-old cannot see as sharply as an 18-year-old. The goal is for the patient to be 20/happy. This means the best vision for the patient, not the best vision based on a standardized test.

There are patients whose vision is excellent, but have, say, symptoms of dry eye disease. That is excess tearing and watering from tears, and those excess tears are not rich in nutrients. Their eyes are uncomfortable. You can be able to see the chart at 20/20, and have uncomfortable eyes every single day. You can have glaucoma, which is the loss of central or peripheral vision due to a whole host of reasons, often including elevated intraocular pressure. It's often called the silent disease of sight because, except in the most extreme cases, there's no pain, symptoms, or other things noticed with glaucoma loss, and you can lose your vision in one eye, while your other eye is seeing 20/20. Because your eyes work in stereo (i.e., they work together) you might not even realize it.

<u>Case Study</u>

The coauthor of this book, Mark Prussian, has been wearing multifocal lenses (bifocal lenses) since his early 30s, and he hasn't been able to see chalkboards since second grade. As a child, Prussian had myopia with astigmatism, and as an adult the diagnosis changed to presbyopia with astigmatism. If LASIK were right for him (it isn't because his corneas are too thin to perform laser surgery), he would be thrilled—assuming his eyes were otherwise healthy—with 20/40, 20/60, or maybe even 20/80 vision. With good intermediate vision, such as viewing the computer screen at his desk, and good distance vision for driving, he would be ecstatic. Prussian states that being able to attend an indoor cycling class or yoga practice without his glasses slipping down his nose would make him 20/Happy regardless of whether 20/20 vision would be achieved.

For some, like Prussian, only needing to wear reading glasses for up-close reading after LASIK would render the procedure a complete success. But for others, needing any correction after LASIK would cause disappointment; it depends on one's goals. That is why it is so important for the patient and the surgeon to agree, preferably in writing, on the vision goal prior to LASIK surgery.

On the other hand, there are people who do special precise work, like airplane model developers or detailed CAD designers like bridge engineers, who are at a computer screen all day, and they may achieve 20/20 or better after LASIK but are totally unhappy because they were expecting—or simply hoping—that what would happen is that LASIK would somehow erase the effects of aging on the eye. LASIK doesn't do that. LASIK can bring you to, in most cases, really good or even perfect visual acuity, but it cannot make your eyes younger again. LASIK does not give you superpowers, nor does it reverse aging. For the most experienced surgeons, 20/Happy rather than 20/20 is the goal.

A disappointed patient is often one who the LASIK surgeon tries to say no to because their vision is already good. Maybe this person just needs a slight correction with glasses or contact lenses for reading or doesn't even need to wear glasses more than an hour or two a day, and now the patient wants to be able to read a book without reading glasses. This person has unrealistic expectations because their vision is good, but the patient is looking for perfection through surgery. They're pretty close to perfect as is. This person had unrealistic expectations without an agreement of postoperative vision with their LASIK surgeon, so now they have unmet expectations and frustration. Often, full-service ophthalmology practices, where eye surgeons perform LASIK regularly, will rightfully reject such potential patients. A great question to ask your LASIK surgeon is what percentage of potential patients they reject.

WHO IS A GOOD CANDIDATE FOR LASIK?

While millions of people have reported a great deal of satisfaction with LASIK eye surgery, it is not right for everyone. In general, individuals who undergo LASIK are able to achieve at least 20/25 vision. This works well for most activities and is acceptable for most people, but it should be understood that you might still need glasses for reading or driving at night as you grow older.

The results you achieve from LASIK will vary based on a number of factors, including your refractive error, which we'll discuss in more detail later on. Individuals with mild nearsightedness usually experience the most success with this procedure. By comparison, people who have a high degree of farsightedness or nearsightedness in addition to astigmatism may have less predictable results. Laser eye surgery tends to be most appropriate for patients who have no unusual vision problems and who have a moderate degree of refractive error.

There are certain conditions that can cause poor surgery outcomes or possible complications:

- Any eye disease that causes progressive vision deterioration
- Thin corneas
- Eye infections
- Lid disorders or eye injuries
- Dry eyes
- Large pupils
- Glaucoma
- Age-related eye changes
- Cataracts
- Diabetic eye disease

Additionally, LASIK may not be appropriate for you if you have fairly good vision. If you are able to see well enough that you only require glasses or contacts part time, you may find that the improvement offered by surgery is not worth the associated risks.

YOUR OVERALL HEALTH

It's also important to consider your overall health in determining whether you are a suitable candidate for LASIK. Certain conditions, such as being under 18 years of age, that are not even related to your eyes can increase surgical risks or make your surgery outcomes less predictable. Health conditions that might make you less suitable as a LASIK candidate including the following:

- Pregnant or nursing
- Any condition or disease that affects your immune system and might make you more prone to infections, such as HIV, rheumatoid arthritis, autoimmune disorders, or lupus
- Diabetes
- Taking an immunosuppressive medication
- Depression
- Chronic pain conditions, such as irritable bowel syndrome, migraines, fibromyalgia, etc.

If you have any of the following conditions, you should also make your surgeon aware of it, as these conditions can affect your surgery or recovery:

- Lazy eye
- Muscle imbalance
- Severe dry eyes
- Previous eye surgery or injury
- Keloid scarring
- Back problems
- Claustrophobia
- Psychological problems

REALISTIC EXPECTATIONS

It is important that you have realistic expectations regarding the outcome of your surgery.

Although some of our LASIK patients start out in glasses, the person who is the best LASIK candidate is typically wearing contact lenses now and wants to see better. Some people just want to simplify their life by not having to deal with contact lenses or glasses. They're also, typically, somewhere between age 20 and 59.

DO YOU HAVE STABLE VISION?

It's also important to consider whether your vision is stable. For instance, if you have myopia, it's possible that your vision might change, which would result in periodic changes to your glasses or contact lenses prescription. For this reason, you would need to be at least 18 years old in order to qualify for LASIK.

There are also certain medications and conditions that can result in temporary fluctuations to your vision, including breast feeding, pregnancy, and taking any type of steroid drugs. If that is the case, you should wait until your vision has stabilized. To qualify for LASIK surgery, you would need to have a contact lens or eyeglasses prescription that has remained stable for a minimum of one year.

YOUR AGE

Age is often a big factor when considering LASIK. As previously mentioned, anyone who is under the age of 18 would usually be disqualified from having LASIK eye surgery. This is because refractive errors have typically not stabilized by this age. The FDA has approved LASIK for people who are at least 18 years of age, but young adults are often cautioned to wait until vision is stable (doesn't change on a yearly basis) before considering LASIK.

On the flip side, some middle-aged persons and almost all seniors are not ideal candidates for LASIK. This is because the eyes begin to change around age 40. This is a condition known as presbyopia, which can make it difficult for people to see objects within an arm's length. LASIK cannot correct this condition. Also, as individuals grow older, certain eye diseases such as glaucoma and cataracts can prevent them from being good candidates for this procedure.

While not everyone over age 40 is completely pleased with LASIK as a stand-alone procedure, there are many laser vision correction options for people over 40. Doctors can correct one eye for near and one eye for distance, called monovision, which gives the stereo effect of wearing multifocal lenses. Other changes to the way the laser is used can reduce astigmatism, and there are even surgical implants that may be better options than using a laser to correct for reading vision. The surgical implants, or other inlays, are usually done in the ophthalmologist's office at the same time as the laser vision correction.

IS IT WORTH THE MONEY TO BUY LASIK IF YOU'RE OVER 40?

As the eye ages, cataracts develop. This most often requires surgery at around age 65. The cataract is completely independent of the benefits of LASIK. Some long-term contact lens wearers are thrilled to find that LASIK technology has improved to the point where having LASIK in your 40s or 50s can give you 5 or 10 years of really good vision before cataracts form. However, this group is split among their opinions on the price. For some contact lens wearers in their 40s or 50s, however, they believe that purchasing LASIK is a great value compared to the possibility of spending another decade in contact lenses. For many glasses wearers, they feel the cost of surgery isn't a good value when cataracts are going to negate the effects of LASIK. Ultimately, the choice is up to you.

WHAT'S THE SIZE OF YOUR PUPIL?

In determining whether you are a suitable candidate for LASIK, it's important to consider the size of your pupil. This is because larger pupils can cause interference with surgical results. Patients with larger pupils have a tendency to experience side effects following their surgery. These are some of the common side effects:

- Halos
- Glares

- Double vision
- Starbursts

Such effects can be quite debilitating and even prevent patients from being able to drive in bad weather or at night. For this reason, your pupil size will be measured during your initial consultation and exam and will assist in determining whether you are a good candidate for this procedure.

THICK OR THIN CORNEAS?

Another common factor that disqualifies many people from being good candidates for LASIK is the thickness of their corneas. Generally speaking, if you have thin corneas, you would not qualify for laser eye surgery. When LASIK is performed on thin corneas, complications can arise. Every situation is different, but in some cases, if you do not qualify for LASIK because of thin corneas, you, along with your surgeon, might find that PRK is a better option.

CORNEAL SCARRING

Individuals may also be disqualified from LASIK if they have corneal scarring. This type of scarring could result from previous eye surgery or an eye injury. The presence of corneal scarring can be determined during a presurgical eye exam.

WILLINGNESS TO FOLLOW THROUGH WITH PRE-SURGERY AND POSTSURGERY RESPONSIBILITIES

While laser eye surgery has undergone a number of advancements in just the last few years, it's still important to understand that you, as a patient, will have a number of important responsibilities regarding preparing for your procedure and recovering from surgery. For instance, if you wear contact lens, you may need to stop wearing them for one to two weeks prior to your surgery. You will also need to make arrangements for postsurgery transportation. Additionally, you will need to comply with follow-up eye exams and a medication schedule. Doing so will help determine how well your eyes heal following the surgery.

WHAT IS A REFRACTIVE VISION ERROR?

Refractive errors refer to vision problems that occur when the eye's shape prevents you from focusing as well as you should. This could be the length of the eyeball—it could be longer or shorter than it should be. It might also be changes in the shape of the cornea or even aging of the lens that create problems.

There are four major refractive errors:

- Myopia
- Hyperopia
- Presbyopia
- Astigmatism

The most common symptom that many people experience with refractive vision errors is blurred vision. Other symptoms might include haziness, double vision, headaches, halos or glare around bright lights, eye strain, headaches, or squinting.

According to the Vision Council of America, approximately 75 percent of adults use some sort of vision correction. About 64 percent of them wear eyeglasses, and about 11 percent wear contact lenses, either exclusively, or with glasses.[1]

WHAT CAUSES REFRACTIVE ERRORS?

All refractive errors are caused by light that does not bend or refract as it should when it strikes the eye. Individuals who are nearsighted have problems seeing things far away. Conversely, farsighted individuals have trouble seeing objects up close. With an astigmatism, you have an oblong (football-shaped) eye which creates multiple points of focus and therefore causes objects to appear blurry.

Children usually have clear up-close and distance vision. Beginning around adolescence, some people may develop a refractive error and require corrective lenses. Between adolescence and adulthood, the

---

[1] glasscrafter.com

prescription for such lenses may change. Refractive errors usually stabilize after adulthood. Once many people hit middle age, however, they may develop presbyopia, which occurs when the natural lens in the eye is no longer as flexible as it once was. As a result, you may not be able to see as well up close as you once did.

MYOPIA

Myopia, or nearsightedness, is commonly caused by blurred vision. It could be mild, moderate, or severe. Persons who are nearsighted may find that objects in the distance are blurry and seem out of focus. When trying to see objects at a distance clearly, you might frown or squint. Myopia is usually not caused by a condition or disease. Instead, it occurs as a result of natural changes that occur within the shape of the eyeball. This can result in problems related to the way that light rays enter the eye in order to focus in front of the retina. Light should focus directly on the retina.

SYMPTOMS OF MYOPIA

The primary symptom of myopia is blurred vision when viewing objects at a distance. If you are able to see well enough to read up close but you find it hard to see objects farther away, you may have myopia. For instance, you might have noticed that you may have difficulty seeing words on television or a movie screen.

Nearsightedness usually occurs in childhood sometime between the ages of 6 and 12. The eyeballs continue to grow during the teen years. As a result, myopia may worsen quickly. It's not uncommon for teens to need new glasses at least once a year. Myopia usually ceases getting worse by the time you are age 20 and begins to stabilize.

HYPEROPIA

Hyperopia refers to being farsighted. This means you are able to see objects at a distance better than objects up close. In this refractive error, light rays do not bend correctly in order to properly transmit images to the brain. Farsightedness often runs in families.

SYMPTOMS OF HYPEROPIA

Symptoms of farsightedness includes eye strain, headaches, and problems focusing on nearby objects. Contact lenses, eyeglasses, or refractive surgery can help to correct hyperopia.

ASTIGMATISM

If you have an astigmatism, it means that your eye is not completely round. Most people have some degree of astigmatism though normal eyeballs are quite round. Therefore, light is able to come into the eye and bend in an even manner. This gives you clear vision. If your eyeball is not perfectly round, light may bend more in one direction than in another direction. As a result, only part of an object will be in focus. This may mean that objects viewed at a distance appear wavy and blurry.

Most people with an astigmatism are born with it. There is not an exact known cause at this time. Astigmatism can also result from eye disease or eye injury. While many people believe that you can develop an astigmatism from reading in low light or sitting too close to the TV, that is just a myth.

SYMPTOMS OF ASTIGMATISM

The most common symptom of an astigmatism is blurry vision. It can be easy to think you are simply experiencing eyestrain or fatigue, but blurry vision is usually the first major indication of an astigmatism. Astigmatism is usually diagnosed through an eye exam.

HIGHER-ORDER ABERRATIONS

A higher-order aberration (HOA) is a more complex type of vision error. If you have been told by an eye doctor that you have an HOA, you might wonder what the impact would be on your vision. HOAs include spherical aberration, coma, defocus, trefoil, and other unfamiliar names. These types of aberrations can result in vision problems that include glare, problems seeing at night, starburst patterns, blurring, halos, and double vision.

Basically, a higher-order aberration is a type of distortion that occurs when light is passed through the eye because of irregularities in the eye. For instance, if the crystalline lens and curvature of the cornea are abnormal, the wavefront of light that passes through the eye might be distorted.

Because most people do not have perfect eyes, most people have, at the very least, a slight HOA. There is usually no need to be concerned if you have been diagnosed with a HOA, unless it seems to cause significant vision problems. In some cases, serious HOAs might occur as a result of eye disease, trauma, or surgery.

HOAs can also be caused by cataracts that cloud the natural lens of the eye. If you suffer from dry eyes, the eye's tear film could be diminished, which might also cause aberrations.

DIAGNOSING HIGHER-ORDER ABERRATIONS

HOAs are usually identified according to the types of distortions that occur when a wavefront of light passes through the eye. A wavefront exam can help to detect the amount of aberrations that may be present and causing vision problems.

WHICH TYPES OF VISION ERRORS CAN LASIK CORRECT?

- Nearsightedness
- Farsightedness
- Astigmatism

WHY CONSIDER GETTING LASIK?

For many people, the decision to have LASIK comes down to the ability to enjoy a changed lifestyle. For readers, athletes, nature lovers, and anyone else who enjoys an active lifestyle, LASIK can help quite a bit. For example, for anyone who enjoys photography, having contact lenses or glasses up close to the eye and the camera, can create difficulties.

Earlier in this chapter you met Mark Prussian, coauthor of this book, board-certified healthcare administrator, and CEO of a large ophthalmology practice for almost all of his career. Prussian's need for glasses started in second grade. It was also around this time that his love of baseball began. In an ironic twist of fate, playing little league and being so nearsighted, Prussian's family was most concerned with whether he would break his glasses, rather than how well he hit the ball or how well he fielded balls to third base. Soon, Prussian was moved to the outfield. Prussian's time as a Little Leaguer ended soon after that. He has expended his continuing enthusiasm for baseball as an avid fan rather than playing the sport he loves so. For Prussian's entire eye care career, eyeglasses, contact lenses, and even LASIK have been a paid employee benefit, but as a child, the cost associated with replacement of glasses created a barrier to his participation in his favorite sport.

Later, Prussian entered the healthcare administration field and now has been running a large eye care practice for an extended period of time. Regardless, he is not a candidate for LASIK, even though he's been educating, promoting, and helping people achieve their best possible vision with LASIK for quite some time. Prussian's corneas are too thin to yield good post-LASIK vision results. Also, the topography of Prussian's eyes has more troughs and valleys than most people's eyes. Through real-life examples, like that of the coauthor of this book, it is important to understand that not everyone is an ideal candidate for LASIK.

LASIK can also save a tremendous amount of frustration. People who are outside and inside, especially during the heat of summer, may find they can particularly benefit from LASIK. If you've ever worn glasses on a really hot and humid day, your glasses will fog up when you get out of an air-conditioned car. If you then you go into an air-conditioned building, your glasses will fog up again. Needless to say, this can be very frustrating. LASIK can eliminate those problems.

Additionally, LASIK can help you save time in your day. Some contact lens wearers spend between 10 and 15 minutes a day inserting contact lenses, removing contact lenses, ordering more contact lenses, buying solutions, adding wetting eye drops, and so forth. With LASIK, you get all of that time back to yourself. Say you're traveling; just having LASIK makes all that so much more convenient. The same is also true for people who enjoy camping or hunting and who want to be free from glasses or contact lenses for a night or a weekend or something like that—it's a savings of time and effort.

Having LASIK can also help to eliminate quite a bit of fear. Imagine: you are so nearsighted that you couldn't find your glasses without wearing your glasses, and you're in a hotel room. You're startled in the middle of the night, and they drop underneath the bed. It's an unfamiliar room you're in. There is nothing more frightening or worrisome than wondering how you're going to find your glasses when you're not familiar with the room. What happens many times with people who are so nearsighted is that they step on their glasses and break them while they are looking for them. All that goes away with LASIK.

LASIK can also be cheaper than contact lenses and far less expensive than glasses. For most people, there are three options for contact lens. One is worn for medical indications. Then, you've got your extended wear, which can be worn for two weeks to a month or so. They are supplied in intervals of two weeks or months. Then, you've got your daily disposable contact lenses. The daily disposables are the ones that do not need any solution, do not need any cleaning or sterilization. When you take them out of your eye, you throw them away in the garbage. This is not only expensive, but also bad for the environment because it comes in a foil pack. You're using and creating lots of trash, and landfill waste. Also, it's not good for your eyes in any of those circumstances. Sleeping in them overnight is a really bad idea. Your eyes need oxygen to be healthy, and the contact lens blocks the clear passage of oxygen. Daily disposable wear contact lenses cost about $1–$3 a day. That comes to about $365–$1,000 per year.

LASIK is also more affordable than continually wearing glasses. A lot of the cost of the glasses is the frame. If you're buying designer frames, and you're buying a high-end lens that protects you from the sun, this could easily be a $300 to $1,000 purchase. If you're fashion-conscious and like to change your glasses style every year, you've got that cost on top of it. People who buy glasses and change their frames every year often spend what amounts to $5 a day on those designer frames. For many people, the option of being glasses-free is a much better choice.

DEBUNKING LASIK MYTHS

There are numerous myths about laser eye surgery. If you are considering having LASIK, it's important to separate fact from myth.

Myth: Contact Lenses Are Safer Than LASIK

Truth: This is not the case. A study performed in 2009 by McGee and Mathers found that risk of vision loss with daily-wear contact lenses and LASIK was about the same. While rigid gas permeable contact lenses are considered safer than laser eye surgery,

LASIK is actually safer than daily-wear soft contact lenses in situations that are more favorable for LASIK.

Myth: LASIK Increases the Risk of Halos and Glare

Truth: Studies have shown that the risk of halos and glare was reduced with patients three months after laser eye surgery was performed. Another study found that nearly 90 percent of pilots landing aircraft at night found that their night vision was actually better following laser eye surgery without glasses compared to their night vision wearing glasses before having LASIK.

Myth: Dry Eye Is Common After LASIK

Truth: Some people do report mild to moderate dry eye after LASIK. Between 1 and 3 percent of patients reported severe dry eye; however, studies show that patient satisfaction from LASIK is still extremely high, even for those suffering from some form of dry eye.

Myth: LASIK Is Painful

Truth: LASIK is very fast and basically pain-free. Prior to treatment, numbing drops are applied to the patient's eyes. This helps limit any discomfort the patient might experience. Most patients only experience a slight moment of pressure as the corneal flap is created. In fact, most patients are actually surprised at how fast the surgery is.

Patients who feel somewhat anxious prior to the procedure can always ask to receive a mild sedative prior to the surgery.

Myth: LASIK Is Only Appropriate for Nearsighted Patients

Truth: In the beginning, LASIK was only performed on nearsighted patients. Since that time, a lot has changed. Now, LASIK can correct a number of refractive errors, including farsightedness, nearsightedness, and astigmatism.

Myth: Patients Who Have LASIK Can Go Blind

Truth: There are no recorded cases of any patient who has had LASIK going blind following surgery. LASIK actually only treats the eye's surface layer to reshape the cornea. Complications occur rarely, and any complications that do occur usually subside over time.

Myth: LASIK Is Unaffordable

Truth: Over the years, the cost of LASIK has decreased quite a bit with the improvement of technology. Now that this form of treatment is more common, there are also financing plans available that can make the procedure even more affordable.

Myth: LASIK Effects Only Last for a Few Years

Truth: Most LASIK treatments offer permanent correction for refractive errors. It is only rare that nearsightedness, astigmatism, or farsightedness return after a patient has LASIK performed. Patients who do experience any form of regression may be able to receive an enhancement surgery. It should be understood that patients may still be at risk for experiencing age-associated vision changes. Such changes may include macular degeneration or cataracts.

Myth: There's a Long Recovery Time with LASIK

Truth: Most patients notice improved vision within about 15 minutes after their procedure is complete. Full LASIK recovery can be expected within 24 hours. There is generally no significant downtime.

Myth: Everyone Is Eligible for LASIK

Truth: As it turns out, not everyone is a good candidate for LASIK. There could be many reasons why you might not be a good candidate for LASIK, including having thin corneas or a medical condition that might interfere with your recovery. Also, while LASIK can correct many refractive errors, some vision problems cannot be corrected with LASIK.

As the eye ages, cataracts develop. This often requires surgery at around age 65. The cataract is completely independent of the benefits of LASIK. Some long-term contact lens wearers are thrilled to find that LASIK technology has improved to the point where having LASIK in your 40s or 50s can give you 5 or 10 years of really good vision before cataracts form. However, this group is split among their opinions on the price. For most contact lens wearers in their 40s or 50s, they believe that purchasing LASIK is a great value compared to the possibility of spending another decade in contact lenses.

For many glasses wearers, they feel the cost of surgery isn't a good value when cataracts are going to eventually negate the effects of LASIK. Ultimately, the choice is up to you.

THE INITIAL CONSULTATION

The first step in having LASIK performed is scheduling an evaluation. This is also known as a consultation. During this appointment, your candidacy for laser eye surgery will be evaluated. Following a thorough discussion and eye exam, a determination will be made about whether laser eye surgery is appropriate for you. The best procedure for your needs can then be recommended, based on your eye exam results.

What Happens during the Consultation?

When you go to the LASIK center for your first consultation, you should expect the following:

- You will meet with your LASIK counselor and technician to discuss the procedure and answer any questions you may have.

- The LASIK technician will record and document your medical and eye care condition. The technician will also perform a refraction vision check and see how dry your eyes may be.
- The technician then performs many digital diagnostic tests to check the shape and thickness of your cornea, which allows the surgeon to have as much predictive analysis as possible about your surgical outcome
- Then you'll meet with your LASIK surgeon. The doctor will review your tests, examine your eyes and review the results with you so that you and the surgeon can jointly decide how to achieve the best vision outcome.
- Lastly, you will again talk with the surgical counselor who will explain the LASIK journey from beginning to end. Many patients choose their surgery date at this visit and schedule postop visits as well.

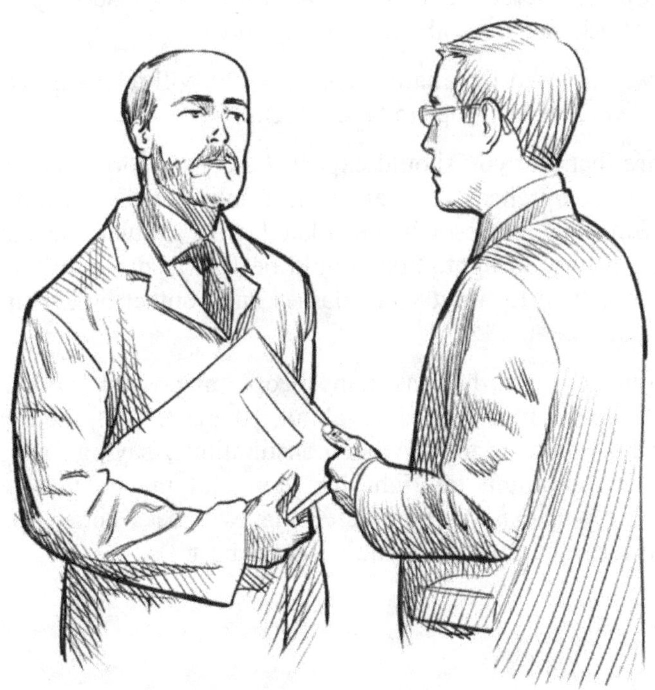

MEASUREMENT OF PUPIL, TEAR DUCT FUNCTION, AND WAVEFRONT ANALYSIS

This test is important because some patients with large pupils may not be good candidates for LASIK due to the risk of possible side effects, such as halos or glare. Your tear duct production will also be checked. Patients who have naturally dry eyes could be at risk for complications following the procedure.

In some cases, a custom wavefront analysis may also be performed. With this analysis, a blueprint can be created to customize your vision correction. While a traditional eye exam can be subjective in nature because it's based on a patient's answers and how he or she thinks they see, wavefront technology provides a more objective analysis of your vision. This is because it is based on the way in which the light travels through the eye.

After your eye exam is finished, the results of your tests will be discussed with you along with your candidacy for laser eye surgery. If you are considered a good candidate for laser eye surgery, you will be able to ask questions about the procedure.

Drops will be used for dilating your eyes. It will take approximately 20 minutes for these drops to take effect.

Be aware that that you should expect the consultation and eye exam to be very comprehensive. Plan for it to take between two and three hours. Since your eyes will be dilated, you should also anticipate some sensitivity to light. You should be fine to drive on the day of your exam. Plan to bring your glasses and contact box with you to your appointment.

While our goal is to help as many people as possible with LASIK, many surgeons report sending about 10 percent of their patients away who come in for LASIK consultations, saying "Glasses or contact lenses might be right for you, and maybe in the future technology will exist or be created that will be a better option for you, but for right now, what you've got is best."

UNDERCORRECTION

Every patient is unique. As a result, every eye is unique and might respond to the healing process differently. Your individual treatment plan will be based on average healing responses of individuals who have undergone LASIK in the past. The software behind wavefront-guided LASIK continues to build each surgeon's database of actual LASIK results, so that undercorrection is less likely to happen as surgeon experience grows. Therefore, having LASIK with a surgeon who has performed at least a few thousand LASIK procedures is the best way to prevent undercorrection.

The chances of an overcorrection or undercorrection being created tend to be higher when treating higher correction levels. Generally speaking, both undercorrection and overcorrection can be treated with a retreatment or enhancement procedure. Patients who have either very steep or thin corneas or those with high degrees of refractive errors might not be good candidates for enhancements. For this reason, it is important for patients to discuss their potential eligibility for enhancements or retreatments. In situations in which a retreatment or enhancement is not an option, contact lenses or glasses can be used to adjust the undercorrection or overcorrection successfully.

ASSESSING VISUAL SATISFACTION POST-LASIK

Multiple factors could affect a patient's satisfaction following laser eye surgery including the following:

- Whether you are farsighted, nearsighted, or have an astigmatism
- The health and characteristics of your corneas
- Age
- The severity of your refractive error
- The strength of your eyeglass prescription
- Your own personal expectations

While LASIK can correct high degrees of nearsightedness, astigmatism, and farsightedness with success, young people who have mild astigmatism or nearsightedness typically experience the best outcomes.

The expectations you have prior to your laser vision surgery will also play a critical role in how satisfied you are with your procedure. It should be kept in mind that the goal of laser eye surgery is to decrease the amount you depend on glasses while helping you see relatively well without the need for corrective lenses. Results can vary from one person to another.

While most people who have had laser vision surgery report seeing better than they did with contact lenses or eyeglasses prior to the surgery, not everyone is the same.

WHEN MIGHT LASIK ENHANCEMENTS BE NEEDED?

There is no reason to panic if your vision is not immediately clear following laser vision surgery. When evaluating your visual acuity following laser vision surgery, it is important to be patient. Most people are able to see much better without eyeglasses the day after the procedure, but it is not uncommon for vision to fluctuate for up to several weeks following the surgery. Your vision will need to be monitored by your eye doctor for several weeks to several months following the procedure.

Some people do feel uncomfortable driving or during other visual tasks following their procedure. It is important that you tell your eye doctor if this happens. You may need to have new eyeglasses prescribed to wear part time until your vision has improved and stabilized. If you notice that your vision still seems blurry three months after your procedure, it is possible that you might need an enhancement. It will be necessary for your corneas to be reevaluated using the same techniques as prior to your first procedure in order to determine whether you are a good candidate for an enhancement. Among the most important factors is whether your corneas are thick enough to allow for a second procedure.

HOW DOES AN ENHANCEMENT COMPARE WITH A PRIMARY PROCEDURE?

LASIK enhancements differ from the original procedure because a flap does not need to be created. Instead of a laser being used to create the corneal flap, specialized tools will instead be used to re-lift the flap, which only takes a couple of minutes. An excimer laser can then be used to reshape your cornea. In most enhancements, only minimal reshaping of the cornea is necessary. Patients will usually need to follow the same postop instructions as were provided for their primary procedure. It is crucial that you follow those instructions in order to ensure a good outcome and reduce the risk of infection.

RISK OF CORNEAL FLAP IRREGULARITIES

Small wrinkles known as striae can occur within the corneal flap following laser eye surgery. These wrinkles do not usually interfere with vision. Additional treatment is not typically required. In some cases, the striae may be significant enough that the patient's visual acuity is decreased. When this happens, it may be necessary to lift the flap so that it can be irrigated and then put back into place. Generally speaking, this procedure, which is very quick, is sufficient to correct the complication.

CAUSES OF FLAP IRREGULARITIES

There are numerous reasons that could cause striae or flap irregularities. Such irregularities tend to be more common when the procedure is performed on very nearsighted eyes. Patients who rub their eyes before the flap has properly bonded may also be more at risk for developing subtle striae. This risk can be avoided by not rubbing your eyes for several weeks following the procedure. If suction is lost during the creation of the flap, complications may also occur.

Other potential complications that might occur with LASIK including the following:

- Irregular or incomplete corneal flaps

- Flaps that are too thin or too small
- Buttonholes (small tears or holes in the center of the flap)
- Free caps (flaps without a hinge)

HALOS AND VISION GLARE

Decreased contrast sensitivity and vision glare are also common side effects that can occur within the first few days following the procedure. In most cases, these problems diminish over time after the surgery. Some LASIK patients report vision glare as auras or halos around lights, such as tail lights or headlights at night. In some cases, patients may experience streaks or starburst around streetlights.

HOW PUPILS CAN AFFECT VISION GLARE

Pupil size can affect the quality of your vision following the procedure. Patients with large pupils may experience more halos than those with smaller pupils. Due to the fact that pupils dilate in dim lighting, some patients may notice they experience reduced vision quality in dark environments.

It is also not uncommon for some people to experience dry eyes following their procedure. This is particularly common during the first few weeks while the corneas are still healing. Patients who have preexisting dry eye conditions should be fully evaluated prior to their surgery. Some patients who have a preexisting dry eye problem may find that their eyes are worse following the procedure.

These are some possible dry eye symptoms following LASIK:

- Excess tears and watery eyes
- A gritty, sandy feeling in the eyes
- Burning sensation
- Feeling as though something is in your eye
- Sensitivity to light
- A heavy feeling to the eyes
- Pain in the eyes

It is thought that one reason why some people experience dry eye symptoms following LASIK is because some of the corneal nerves may be disturbed during the creation of the corneal flap. This can be a problem because the corneal nerves are responsible for providing feedback to the tear glands. As a result, there is a reduction in the flow of tears of the eyes. Once healing has taken place, the corneal endings will usually regenerate, which means tear volume will return gradually and dry eye symptoms will disappear.

CHAPTER 3

A COMPLETE GUIDE TO THE LASIK PROCEDURE

Today, LASIK is the most commonly performed laser eye surgery for treating astigmatism, hyperopia, and myopia. As discussed previously, LASIK reshapes the cornea, making it possible for light to enter the eye so it can be focused onto the retina properly, thus producing clearer vision. Generally speaking, the procedure is relatively pain-free and can be performed quickly. As a result, patients are able to enjoy improved vision without the need for contact lenses or eyeglasses. Many patients report they are able to enjoy clearer vision within 24 hours.

> ***LASIK Defined in Just 50 words:*** *LASIK eye surgery is the process of changing the curvature of the cornea to improve and correct how we see. During the procedure, the surgeon cuts a flap on the side of the cornea and peels it back to reveal fresh tissue that an excimer laser shaves away to correct.*

The actual surgical time for the LASIK procedure is only about 15 minutes. When the patient enters the LASIK suite, he or she is positioned on the bed and made comfortable while the computer inputs data specific to the eyes. The time the lasers are functioning are only about five to ten seconds for each eye.

HOW IS LASIK PERFORMED?

If you're considering having laser eye surgery, it's only natural to be curious about how the procedure is actually done. As we discussed earlier, LASIK technology has improved tremendously since it was first introduced. Surgeon now have a multitude of approaches for laser eye surgery.

These are the actual surgeon's steps in LASIK:

- Using the data collected from the digital diagnostic scans of your eye, a treatment plan is created.
- The treatment plan is entered into the computer that powers the femtosecond laser and the excimer laser.
- The surgeon verifies all the data.
- A femtosecond laser is used to create a thin, almost-circular flap in the cornea.
- The surgeon folds back the hinged flap, so that the cornea can be accessed.
- The excimer laser is used to remove precise amounts of corneal tissue.
- This process is then repeated for the second eye.

In the last chapter, we discussed the tests that are conducted prior to laser eye surgery. One of the tests is to evaluate the moistness of your eyes. A precautionary treatment is sometimes used in order to reduce the risk of dry eyes developing following the procedure. An automated instrument known as a corneal topographer is used for measuring the curvature of the front of the eye. A map of the cornea is also created.

With advanced LASIK, which uses wavefront optimized technology, a wavefront analysis is performed. Using a wavefront abberometer, the analysis transmits light waves through the eye, which creates a precise map of any aberrations that may be present in the eye.

DIFFERENT WAYS LASERS CAN BE USED TO RESHAPE THE CORNEA

There are several different ways excimer lasers can be used for reshaping the cornea.

Traditional/Standard

In traditional or standard LASIK, the cornea is reshaped to treat farsightedness, nearsightedness, and astigmatism with lower order aberrations using approximately the same measurements that are used for contacts or glasses. The patient's eyeglass or contact lens prescription is the primary information used for reshaping the cornea. Consequently, two patients who might just happen to have the same prescription would receive about the same corneal shape.

With standard LASIK, it's possible for light rays to focus near or on the retina once the shape of the cornea is changed. Excimer lasers are used to create a cool beam of light that changes the corneal shape. Rather than being directed on the surface cells, the laser light from the excimer laser is directed on the inner part of the cornea. LASIK enjoys a high degree of success because the light beam is directed to the cornea's inner layer. A microkeratome is then used to lift a thin slice of the cornea's top layer. Once the corneal flap has been folded back, the middle section of the cornea is exposed. The flap is then repositioned while the laser emits pulses of light onto the cornea.

If you are having LASIK on an older excimer laser, then you will probably have your flap created using a manual keratome. A manual keratome is essentially a scalpel or blade in a holder that makes cutting into the corneal layer fairly precise. Most modern LASIK centers use a femtosecond laser rather than a manual keratome.

Many patients experience functional vision within a few hours after their advanced LASIK procedure, although it's quite common to experience some watering of the eyes. Some patients may feel as though they have an eyelash in their eye for about two to three hours following the procedure. From that point, patients usually do not experience any pain. There may continue to be some blurriness, but this usually improves significantly after getting a good night's sleep. For persons receiving standard LASIK, vision improvement time varies.

Wavefront Guided

For patients who want to achieve better, sharper vision, a custom wavefront LASIK procedure may an option. Custom wavefront LASIK is also known as wavefront LASIK or custom LASIK. With conventional LASIK surgery, the goal is to recreate the vision correction offered by the patient's eyeglasses or contact lenses prescription. The problem with this is that these prescriptions are not unique. It's possible for thousands of people to have the same prescription.

Due to the fact that everyone's eyes have unique characteristics, conventional technology simply cannot measure those characteristics or determine unique refractive errors. Because of this, people who have the same prescription will actually see with varying degrees of clarity when they undergo standard or traditional laser eye surgery.

With advanced wavefront technology, it's possible to evaluate the unique characteristics of the patient's eyes and achieve a higher degree of personalization and precision.

Custom LASIK utilizes far more detailed information than just the prescription to program the excimer laser so that the patient's eyes can be reshaped to their specific needs during the procedure. Wavefront technology offers two important benefits over traditional LASIK.

Custom wavefront LASIK is much more precise than standard laser eye surgery. To demonstrate how important this is, think about a routine eye exam. During this exam, the doctor uses different lenses, asks you to look at the eye chart and then asks you to tell him whether the first or second lens is clearer. As you have probably experienced, it can be difficult to choose which lens is clearer because they look the same. Every click on the dial for the instrument used to determine your prescription is an extremely small unit of power, representing 0.25 diopter. You might have noticed that your eyeglass prescription features numbers like -1.25 D (diopter) or -1.50 D. This is why.

When custom wavefront LASIK is used, the power of lenses necessary for vision correction is measured in 0.01 diopter. By using a diopter increment rather than 0.25, more precise corrections can be made to evaluate refractive errors. Also, instead of having you decide which lens is clearer, a computer makes the more accurate choice.

Besides the advantage of more precise refractive evaluation, custom wavefront LASIK is also more specific. When your prescription is measured during an eye exam, the doctor evaluates the ability of your eyes to focus light as a whole. In other words, one lens prescription is determined for the entire eye. With custom LASIK, hundreds of separate reference points are gathered on the eye's surface. All of this information is gathered together to produce a detailed map of focusing imperfections. That information can then be used to program the laser to produce a highly personalized vision correction based on the patient's specific needs. The map used in this procedure can help measure distortions that contacts and glasses are not able to correct. Along with being able to treat astigmatism, farsightedness, and nearsightedness, wavefront guided LASIK can help reduce irregular higher-order aberrations that could actually reduce clarity of vision even after any other major refractive errors, such as glare and halo that some patients experience, can be reduced.

Wavefront Optimized

Wavefront optimized LASIK is a treatment pattern that uses all of the benefits of wavefront guided plus superior technology enhancements to create and maintain the round, natural curve of the eye. This helps produce crisp, sharp vision while reducing the likelihood of nighttime halo and glare following the procedure. Detailed measurements of the front of the eye's curvature are used in order to preserve the cornea's natural aspheric shape. By doing so, it's possible to reduce the risk of a certain higher-order abnormalities known as spherical aberration which can also result in halo, glare, and other night vision problems.

An instrument known as an aberrometer is used in custom ablation to create a specialized map known as a wavescan. An aberrometer can measure a number of optical eye properties that simply cannot be measured using a basic eyeglasses fitting. As a result, it's possible to create an optical fingerprint. A computer utilizes all of this data for correcting all optical aberrations during the laser eye surgery procedure.

IS WAVEFRONT OPTIMIZED LASIK BETTER THAN STANDARD LASIK?

Just like with fingerprints, no two treatments that are the same. Results have shown that advanced wavefront optimized LASIK can help patients achieve better vision than with standard LASIK.

It should be noted that while advanced wavefront optimized LASIK does offer a number of benefits for vision correction, not everyone is a suitable candidate for it. A number of factors must be considered in determining which type of LASIK might be appropriate for a patient. These factors include the thickness of the cornea, eyeglasses prescription, and the patient's satisfaction with their vision with glasses. Other considerations are patients who have a very small pupil size or who have a high degree of myopia or astigmatism. Standard or traditional LASIK is still quite effective for patients who may not qualify for advanced LASIK.

EXCIMER LASERS

The field of laser eye surgery has been revolutionized by the use of excimer lasers. Numerous advances have been made in excimer laser technology over the years, thus increasing the efficacy, safety, and predictability of refractive surgery.

The excimer laser was first used for performing laser vision correction in 1987. In 1995, it was approved for use in the United States by the FDA for the correction of nearsightedness. As technology advanced, it has also been approved for treating and farsightedness.

Excimer lasers can also be used to correct astigmatism. This is done by smoothing an irregularly shaped cornea so it has a normal shape. Once the cornea has been reshaped, the flap can then be put back into place. The cornea can then be allowed to heal naturally.

Excimer lasers produce beams of ultraviolet laser lights with multiple properties. An excimer laser's energy is absorbed immediately when it encounters the tissue of the human cornea. Due to the fact that the cornea has a high water content, the laser penetrates only the eye's surface. The corneal surface is vaporized by the excimer laser without resulting in any damage to surrounding tissue. As a result, it's possible to sculpt the surface of the cornea in a precise manner.

FDA AND LASIK

Before any medical device can be sold legally in the United States, approval must be gained from the Food and Drug Administration (FDA). In order to gain approval, evidence must be presented demonstrating that the device is effective and safe. While the sale of excimer lasers is regulated by the FDA, the FDA is also responsible for monitoring its safety. The FDA does not have the authority to regulate or tell doctors what to do or how much can be charged for a particular procedure, nor can it make recommendations for individual clinics, eye centers, or doctors. Additionally, the FDA does not maintain a list of doctors who perform laser eye surgery.

During your consultation, ask your LASIK surgeon the make and model number of the excimer laser and femtosecond laser that will be used during your procedure. Check this using the FDA website (www.fda.gov) to find out when it was approved. Your surgeon should be using laser technology that was recently approved.

HOW EXCIMER LASERS WORK

The excimer laser works by meticulously emitting a cool beam of ultraviolet light to remove corneal tissue. Only a small amount of the cornea is penetrated by the high-energy ultraviolet light pulses. Due to the high level of precision involved, it is possible to remove as little as 0.24 microns of tissue. This is an incredibly small amount of tissue as a single micron is equivalent to one-thousandth of a millimeter.

Excimer lasers are capable of correcting nearsightedness by flattening the cornea. Farsightedness can be corrected by creating a steeper cornea. By smoothing an irregular cornea and giving it a more symmetrical shape, it's possible to correct astigmatism. Once the cornea's surface has been reshaped properly, light rays can focus correctly onto the retina, resulting in clearer vision.

Excimer lasers are controlled by computers programmed to correct specific refractive errors. The pattern and quantity of tissue removal are based on each patient's needs and therefore unique to each individual.

Most excimer lasers also utilize automated eye tracking systems designed to monitor eye movements while ensuring the laser beam stays on target during the procedure. Research has shown that correcting for eye movement during the procedure produces better vision outcomes while decreasing the potential complications of LASIK compared to older excimer lasers that do not utilize eye tracking systems.

BLADELESS LASIK

Patients who are considering LASIK eye surgery may have heard the term "bladeless" and wondered how the procedure is done and whether it might be right for them. In the early days of LASIK, an instrument referred to as a microkeratome was used to cut a thin flap into the cornea. The hinged flap was then lifted to apply laser energy to reshape the cornea. The flap was put back in place to promote healing.

In 1999, another method of creating the corneal flap was introduced. This method uses a form of high-energy laser, known as a femtosecond laser, instead of a blade. Since that time, all-laser blade-free LASIK has been shown to produce far more accurate results in most people.

BLADE VS. BLADELESS LASIK

Some discount laser centers still offer blade LASIK, often as a cost-saving, attention-getting measure. In deciding which type of LASIK procedure is best for your needs, it's important to understand exactly what is involved in each. There is sometimes a misconception that both procedures involve cutting and therefore neither are truly bladeless. In fact, there is no blade used in all-laser LASIK. While procedures involving the use of a microkeratome do involve the use of a blade, they are not riskier than all-laser procedures. However, in most persons, a bladed, or microkeratome, produces less accurate visual results.

If you are considering undergoing LASIK with a blade, and price rather than visual acuity is your main concern, then perhaps choosing a LASIK center offering a microkeratome might be right for you!

As technology has advanced, there are known advantages of using a femtosecond laser combined with an excimer laser to create all-laser LASIK versus LASIK with a blade.

Overall, flap predictability is greater with the use of a laser flap than with a blade flap. Of course, it should be understood that flap complications, although rare, can occur with either blade or bladeless procedures. Ultimately, both procedures involve the use of tools that are only as precise as the surgeon handling them.

There has been some contention that microkeratomes create a flap, known as a meniscus flap, that is thinner in the middle. However, there is no consensus data showing that a flap that features the same thickness in the middle, as well as the outer edges, is any better in terms of quality.

There are also fewer risks of a partial flap being created with a laser than with a microkeratome. According to studies, blade flaps involve a greater risk of HOAs occurring than with laser flaps. Clinical trials have substantiated that this is due to the shape of the flap. Bladeless LASIK also involves an issue of transient light sensitivity. This issue appears to be temporary in nature and can usually be treated successfully with the use of steroid eye drops for a few weeks.

Ultimately, LASIK is incredibly safe, regardless of whether it is performed with a microkeratome or with a bladeless system. However, precision increases with all-laser LASIK.

WHAT IS INVOLVED IN ALL-LASER LASIK EYE SURGERY?

Due to the fewer risks and complications involved in bladeless or all-laser eye surgery, it is frequently considered to be the premium option for corrective eye surgery. Additionally, this form of laser eye surgery sometimes makes the procedure possible for individuals, such as those with thin corneas, who once were not considered good candidates for laser eye surgery.

Surgeons, with the assistance of femtosecond computer technology, are now able to create incredibly small flaps in the cornea. This makes it possible to target the tissue and divide it at the molecular level without impact or heat to the adjacent tissue. As a result, it's possible to create a corneal flap in a much more precise manner than when using the microkeratome blade. Bladeless laser eye surgery also makes it possible for the patient to enjoy a faster healing time due to the surgeon's ability to make a more accurate flap that will reposition itself naturally.

While both traditional and bladeless LASIK have the risk of complications, studies have revealed that bladeless laser eye surgery results in fewer overall complication rates. In fact, the flap structure created by an all-laser procedure may reduce the risk of epithelial growth, which is the growth of cells underneath the flap, creating an irregular corneal surface and vision defects. Studies have also shown that bladeless laser eye surgery may result in a lower risk of dry eye following the procedure as well as the need for fewer enhancements.

TYPES OF BLADELESS LASER EYE SURGERY

Bladeless laser eye surgery was first introduced in the United States in 2001. It was at that time that IntraLase gained approval from the FDA for the first femtosecond laser to be used in laser eye surgery. Since then, many rounds of advancements in laser eye surgery have made those first IntraLase lasers nearly obsolete. The best candidates for this procedure include those with mild to moderate myopia, hyperopia, and/or astigmatism with an adequate amount of corneal thickness. The procedure, including set-up time, takes less than ten minutes per eye and has a typical result of being free of contact lenses or glasses. Prospective patients can expect a recovery time measured in hours for stable vision.

BENEFITS OF FEMTOSECOND LASER LASIK

A femtosecond is essentially an ultra-fast laser with ultra-short pulses of light.

Along with being able to put patients at ease that there will be no blade used on their eyes, bladeless laser eye surgery with the use of a femtosecond laser offers the following benefits:

- Decreased risk of abrasions to the cornea during surgery
- More predictability for the thickness of the corneal flap
- Reduced risk of induced astigmatism following the procedure
- Potential ability to correct higher levels of nearsightedness safely

In addition, the femtosecond laser also provides more options in regards to the shape, orientation, and size of the flap. This allows for a more customized procedure based on each patient's specific needs. With the use of a femtosecond laser, it's possible to create a flap with edges that can fit into place more securely following the procedure. This can potentially reduce the amount of healing time involved as well as reduce the risk of the flap becoming dislocated after the surgery.

DIFFERENT TYPES OF LASERS

For patients who are considering having laser eye surgery performed, it is important to understand there are two major types of higher energy lasers. They are excimer lasers and femtosecond lasers.

Excimer lasers produce an ultraviolet light on a specific wavelength. This wavelength is usually 193 nanometers. That light can then be absorbed by the tissue, which makes it possible to remove or ablate the_tissue from the underlying area of the cornea without running the risk of damaging nearby tissue. Most modern excimer lasers today rely on automated eye-tracking systems in order to monitor movements of the eye during the procedure and ensure the ultraviolet beam stays on target. Various patterns may be used for tracking the eye. Two of the primary types are slit-scanning and spot-scanning lasers.

Since LASIK eye surgery was first approved by the FDA, millions of people have relied on the procedure to improve their vision. Today, LASIK is one of the most frequently performed eye procedures in North America.

WAVEFRONT GUIDED LASERS

Among the most advanced excimer lasers in use today are wavefront guided lasers. These types of laser utilize advanced technology for detecting and correcting corneal flaws that other systems cannot pick up. A detailed wavefront map of the patient's eye is used to guide the procedure. This makes it possible to completely customize the treatment. These types of lasers generally provide patients with clearer, sharper vision.

The femtosecond laser combines wavefront technology to generate incredibly precise results. Rather than using a blade to create the thin flap of tissue, a femtosecond laser produces an infrared light beam for creating the flap.

In some cases, excimer lasers and femtosecond lasers may be used in combination. This combination depends on the patient's specific requirements, including degree of refractive error and pupil size.

USING AN INTEGRATED NETWORK TO GIVE YOU THE BEST POSSIBLE VISION

A superb arrow in the hands of an unskilled archer
will not hit the target.

While there are multiple FDA-approved excimer lasers currently on the market, it's only natural for prospective patients to wonder which type of laser might be best for their surgery. It should be understood that one laser is not necessarily better than another. A variety of factors could affect which laser might be best for your needs, including your pupil size, current vision prescription, the thickness of your cornea, and the degree of your refractive error. Among those factors, pupil size can be critical to the outcome of your procedure. Some vision problems, including glare or halos at night, may occur if the patient's pupil expands in low light beyond the laser treatment zone of the cornea. The size of a patient's pupils can affect the type of laser that is used in the procedure. Choosing a surgeon who has lots of experience using their own laser equipment yields the best results. Further, using a laser system designed to function as an integrated unit is essential, but in some discount LASIK centers, mix-and-match lasers can be found.

UNDERSTANDING ABERRATIONS TREATED BY CUSTOM LASER EYE SURGERY

The distortions treated by laser eye surgery are known as aberrations. Most of these aberrations are responsible for common refractive errors, including astigmatism, nearsightedness, and farsightedness. Optical devices, such as contact lenses and glasses, as well as certain laser eye surgeries, can treat most such lower-order aberrations.

A small percentage of optical aberrations create HOAs, including trefoils, coma, quadrafoils, and diffraction. Only a small portion of the general population experience such HOAs. When these aberrations do occur, they are entirely unique to each patient. In many ways, such aberrations are like a fingerprint. Both coma and spherical aberrations can result in blurry images that tend to be more apparent at night. Additionally, both can create halos around lights as well as double vision and glare. These HOAs, including spherical aberrations, coma, and trefoil are types of an irregular astigmatism that cannot be corrected with the use of contact lenses or eyeglasses. Spherical aberrations cause patients to see halos and starbursts around lights while coma causes patients to see a point of light that is similar to a comet. Trefoil results in the point of light to resemble something similar to the Mercedes Benz symbol. The more irregular the shape of the eye, the higher the order of the aberration.

Wavefront LASIK can be beneficial in treating such aberrations because it offers a measurement of the way in which the eye operates in an integrated optical system. The wavefront device provides the surgeon with a highly detailed refractive map of the eye's pupil. In perfect vision, the eye views a far off target with the light from each point in the object entering the eye in a set of parallel rays. The surface perpendicular to each of those rays is the wavefront. With perfect vision, the wavefront enters the eye from a distant object in a flat wavefront that can be focused down to an incredibly small spot.

When the patient suffers from some form of aberration, light enters the eye differently. For instance, with myopia, when the patient looks at a distant target, the parallel light rays do not focus well onto the retina. Instead, they focus in front of the retina. Consequently, by the time the light actually reaches the retina, it is blurry. The patient is therefore only able to see an object if it is near the eye.

Traditional vision testing is actually similar in many ways to wavefront sensing. The patient is asked which combination of lenses is necessary to ensure the flat wavefront from a distant object is focused in the best possible manner back onto the retina. There are limitations, however. For example, there are some higher-order aberrations that cannot be corrected with simple lenses. A common example of this is coma. In the case of coma, one side of the pupil might be more hyperopic than average while the other size is more myopic than average. This results in blurring, an issue that cannot be corrected with simple lenses.

TREATING HIGHER-ORDER ABERRATIONS

Newer forms of laser systems have become so advanced, it's possible to specifically customize the surgery for every patient in the same way that contact lenses or glasses can be customized. Wavefront technology, in the hands of an experienced surgeon, makes it possible to deliver custom treatments while also measuring for even more complex vision aberrations. For instance, while the traditional laser eye procedure works well for treating lower-order aberrations, such as hyperopia, astigmatism, and myopia, wavefront laser eye surgery is beneficial for treating both lower-order aberrations as well as halos, starbursts, glare, and other higher-order aberrations because it makes it possible to reshape the cornea's surface in a custom manner. For many patients, this is the only viable treatment option.

Whereas traditional laser eye surgery relies on the patient's eyeglasses prescription, custom laser eye surgery relies on the use of wavefront technology to create a map of the patient's eyes in order to determine the most accurate prescription. Interestingly, this technology has even been used by astronomers to adjust telescope optics.

While the wavefront system is shining light into the patient's eye, the light reflects back into the wavefront system, thus providing the surgeon with incredibly detailed information about the patient's eyes. Patients who have severe astigmatism may be advised that advanced LASIK is the best option for their needs due to the ability to measure and treat the patient's prescription more accurately.

In order for the patient to benefit from customized corneal shaping, the higher-order optical aberrations will need to be measured. This is done through precise measurements on a corneal mapping instrument prior to the date of the LASIK laser vision correction. These measurements are then digitally interfaced with a networked laser system, which allows the surgeon to utilize high-speed computerized control in order to direct the laser beam's delivery of energy across the surface of the cornea.

Through the corneal mapping, the surgeon can view the refractive aberrations clearly and accurately in rotating 3D images. This is accomplished by the aberrometer transmitting low-energy laser light into the patient's eye. The light then reflects off the patient's retina and is transmitted back through the cornea and the lens. The aberrometer then captures the outgoing wavefront and measures it to determine relevant aberrations. Those aberrations are then displayed on the screen for the surgeon to view.

That data is then interfaced digitally with the excimer laser system in order to create a corneal ablation that is completely customized to the patient. A high-speed computerized eye tracking method can be used with the excimer laser system to assist the surgeon in the treatment by providing precise delivery of the laser beam. Due to the fact that human eyes make extremely fine jumping movements, known as saccadic movements, on a continual basis, a tracking system is used. These movements are beyond the control of the patient, so the eye tracking system assists the surgeon in scanning the eye extremely fast, thousands of times per second, in fact. Computerized controls can then be used to make microadjustments with extreme precision in order to reposition the laser beam as necessary.

The excimer laser system also uses a cool laser light beam that has a very small width, less than the thickness of a single strand of hair. That beam of light can be moved across the corneal surface quite quickly in a small but overlapping pattern, giving the surgeon the ability to create a smooth corneal shape.

Along with wavefront guided laser eye surgery, another way to correct higher-order aberrations is with wavefront optimized laser eye surgery. Among the most common aberrations seen today is spherical aberration. Wavefront optimized laser eye surgery can be beneficial for correcting this specific type of aberration.

IS WAVEFRONT LASIK RIGHT FOR YOU?

Almost everyone can benefit from wavefront LASIK. Every pair of eyes is unique, and wavefront LASIK achieves the maximum results for customizing your treatment to achieve your personal best vision. While custom laser eye surgery utilizes advanced technology, the real benefit is the improved visual quality. This is particularly true in terms of vision in dark environments or at night.

It should be noted that some patients may not be good candidates for wavefront treatment. Situations in which this might occur include when a patient has a corneal scar or when the patient is not able to relax his or her focusing ability in order for a precise measurement to be obtained. In some cases, the pupil diameter may need to be large enough for the aberrometer to take a proper measurement. If the patient's pupil diameter is not large enough in a low light situation, he or she may not be a suitable candidate for this procedure. If the aberrometer is not able to make precise eye measurements, then the procedure is not a good option for that patient.

IMPROVED GLARE CONTROL AND NIGHT VISION

The way in which the eyes dilate or become larger in low light or dim environments is quite important to the success of laser eye surgery. The pupils dilate in order to allow the maximum amount of light possible to enter the eyes on foggy days, at night, or on overcast days. This must be taken into consideration when determining the laser eye correction necessary for each patient. As previously mentioned, if the optical zone is smaller than the pupil size at its largest, there is a risk that the patient will experience problems with poor night vision, halos around bright objects, and glare. Among the factors to be taken into consideration is the ability to create the largest available optical zone, which can help to practically eliminate night vision and glare problems. Experienced LASIK surgeons with advanced technology have the best opportunities to limit glare and poor night vision for patients.

CHAPTER 4
PREPARING FOR LASIK

To help ensure the best possible outcome for your LASIK treatment, it's important to know what to expect before, during, and immediately after your surgery. This guide has been prepared to help you do exactly that.

PREOPERATIVE CONSIDERATIONS

Be aware that prior to your procedure, your surgeon may prescribe medication you will need to take a few days before your treatment. This is often in the form of eye drops that will need to be applied several days prior to the procedure. It is crucial to the outcome of your procedure that you follow the directions carefully and use as instructed.

On the day of your procedure, you will need to wash your face thoroughly. Please do not come to the LASIK center wearing makeup. It is imperative that any traces of cosmetics be removed before the treatment. Baby shampoo can be used along the lash line to remove all mascara and eyeliner. Do not apply any eye rejuvenation gel or moisturizer around your eyes on the day of the procedure. Do not use any perfume or cologne on the day of the procedure, as the fumes could possibly interfere with the laser beam.

Patients who wear contact lenses will need to stop wearing them prior to their evaluation and procedure. This means that you will need to wear your glasses full-time. The reason for this is contact lenses temporarily change the shape of your cornea. The length of time you need to abstain from wearing your contact lenses will depend on the type of lenses you wear. Leaving out your contact lenses for a period of time will allow your cornea to resume its natural shape. If you wear soft contact lenses, your surgeon will ask that you stop wearing them for two weeks prior to your initial evaluation. Rigid gas permeable (RGP) lenses should not be worn for two to three weeks prior to your initial evaluation.

The measurements taken prior to your procedure help determine the precise amount of corneal tissue that needs to be removed in order to provide you with optimal vision. Measurements will be taken during your initial evaluation and also just before your procedure to make certain those measurements have not changed.

It's important that you tell your surgical team about any past or present medical and eye conditions you may have. You should also advise your team of all medications, including over-the-counter medications, you are currently taking. Also, your surgeon will need to know about any medicines to which you are allergic.

Remember, during your evaluation your surgeon will determine whether you are good candidate for laser eye surgery. You will also have the chance to ask any questions you may have. If there is anything you are uncertain about regarding laser eye surgery, this is an excellent time to ask. Make sure you have allowed yourself enough time to think about the risks as well as the benefits of this procedure. Writing down your questions in advance and having them available during the evaluation will ensure the best use of time by you and your LASIK surgeon.

QUELLING YOUR FEAR OF LASER EYE SURGERY

It's not uncommon for many people to have some fears regarding the procedure. Patients are most relaxed when they are educated and know what to expect. For this reason, it's important to take the time to ensure all of your questions are answered prior to surgery.

Some of the most common fears regarding LASIK include the following:

- Fear of pain either during or after the procedure
- Fear of coming into contact with the laser
- Fear of losing vision
- Fear of the scalpel

- Fear of having one's eyes open during the procedure
- Fear of being awake and feeling the procedure

Some people are so afraid of laser eye surgery that they continue to live with poor vision and never even consider the procedure. The reality is that laser eye surgery is very common and quite safe. Millions of people have been helped by LASIK.

To help eliminate some of your fears regarding laser eye surgery, let's bust some of the most common myths.

LASIK Fear: Pain During the Procedure

Although there are some myths that perpetuate the belief that you will feel pain during the procedure, the truth is that you will not feel anything. While you are conscious during the procedure, mild sedation is used along with numbing drops to keep you calm and comfortable. As a result, you do not have to worry about feeling anything beyond a slight pressure. There is no pain. It only takes about five minutes on average to complete the treatment for each eye.

LASIK Fear: Losing Vision

Some people do not consider laser eye surgery because they are afraid they will go permanently blind. The FDA reports there have been no instances of blindness as a result of laser eye surgery. Any vision issues that occur following laser eye surgery can usually be corrected with treatment. Dry eyes, not the loss of vision, is the most common complication following LASIK, and even this happens in far fewer than 1 percent of LASIK patients.

LASIK Fear: Fear of Coming into Contact with the Laser

This is a common concern for many people, and it is certainly understandable. While a laser is involved in LASIK, it is only used for removing corneal tissue. Both the femtosecond laser, which creates the flap, and the excimer laser, which treats the eye, only come into contact with each eye for a few seconds. You should not be concerned that your surgery will be a failure if you move your eye or blink during the treatment. The equipment used is highly sophisticated and includes an eye tracking system that will follow the movement of your eye. This means your surgeon is able to match the pulses of the laser to the movement of your eye. Even if you move your eye, your surgeon can still successfully complete your treatment. As a result, there should be no concerns about blinking during your procedure.

LASIK Fear: Fear of the Scalpel

By choosing a surgeon who uses both a femtosecond and excimer laser, you will be working with a surgeon who performs blade-free LASIK. If you choose a surgeon who does not use all-laser LASIK, you should ask your surgeon why he or she feels a scalpel is a suitable substitute for a laser.

LASIK Fear: Fear of Feeling the Treatment

While you will be conscious during the procedure, your surgeon will use numbing eye drops and a mild sedative to help you relax. This also helps block any sensation of pain, so you should only feel some pressure and no pain at all.

LASIK Fear: Use of Anti-Anxiety Medication and Numbing Eye Drops

Patients are often given a mild anti-anxiety medication prior to their surgery. This is to help ease any nervousness or tension you may experience during the procedure. It is important that you be able to participate in the procedure and follow the surgeon's instructions.

A member of your LASIK surgical team will also apply several eye drops. These numbing drops are used to ensure that you experience the least amount of discomfort possible during the procedure.

THE DAY OF SURGERY

What to Wear

It is a good idea to wear something warm and comfortable, as many people find the laser treatment room to be somewhat cool. You may also bring a sweater or light jacket if you are concerned that you might be cold. Since you will have shields over your eyes following the procedure, do not wear anything that will need to be pulled over your head. You will also need to remove any jewelry before your procedure.

Payment

Laser vision correction is a cosmetic, elective cash-payment procedure. Many LASIK centers require payment or financial arrangements up to a week in advance. Advanced LASIK centers will not be asking you to make payment arrangement on the day of your LASIK procedure, as this will have been handled in advance.

Preoperative Care

Prior to your procedure, you will need to follow some preoperative care instructions:

- Make sure that you have arranged for transportation for the day of your procedure. You will not be able to drive yourself home following your treatment.
- You should be prepared to take medications and/or drops following your procedure. You will need to do so at regular intervals.
- Be aware that while the actual surgery only takes a few minutes, you should plan to be at the center for between one and two hours.
- On the day of the surgery, plan to eat a light meal prior to your treatment. Avoid drinking excessive amounts of caffeine. Beyond this, there are no dietary restrictions prior to having laser eye surgery. While it is recommended that you have a light meal before your procedure, there is no need to force yourself to eat.
- Contact your surgeon prior to the day of your procedure if you have any medical condition changes. This includes severe colds, fever, and so on. You should also consult with your physician if you are on any medications in case there is any need to make adjustments to your medications.

What Happens during Surgery

When the day of surgery finally arrives, you'll be taken into an exam room where the LASIK team will make sure that all of your questions have been answered and that you are made comfortable. In that exam room, the technician will instill eye drops and you will again meet with the surgeon to verify your measurements and desired outcome. You will have a final opportunity to ask the surgeon any questions you may have.

Next, the LASIK team will walk you to the LASIK suite. There you will lie on your back in a reclining chair and be positioned under the laser system. The LASIK team, which consists of the surgeon and two to three other staff members, will verify the measurements placed into the laser system's computer Your surgeon will be speaking with you, and the LASIK team, during the entire procedure to keep you updated on your progress. An instrument, called a lid speculum, will keep your eyelids open during the procedure.

Next, the femtosecond laser will be used to create the flap. After this, the reclining chair will gently move you about two feet so that you are positioned under the excimer laser.

After the creation of the flap, it is folded back to reveal the stroma or underlying cornea. This allows the surgeon to use the excimer laser to remove the appropriate amount of corneal tissue. The laser utilizes a cool ultraviolet light beam to remove microscopic amounts of tissue to reshape the cornea.

Once the surgeon has put the flap back into place and smoothed the cornea, he or she will then apply a special solution to help the flap refloat for proper placement. The cornea begins sealing itself within just a few minutes. You will then rest in the reclining chair for a few minutes, and then the LASIK team will apply anti-inflammatory and antibiotic drops to your eyes. After this is done, the reclining chair is gently moved about two feet so that it is once again underneath the femtosecond laser and treatment of your second eye can begin.

Immediately after Your Procedure

After your laser eye surgery is completed, you will need to rest for a little while. Be aware that it is quite common to experience an itching or burning sensation following the surgery. You should arrange for someone to drive you to the procedure because you will not be able to drive home. You should not drive until the doctor sees you at your one-day postoperative visit.

You should anticipate some haziness and blurry vision immediately after your procedure. By the next morning, you will notice the clarity of your vision improve. You may also notice that your eyes are sensitive to light. Some patients report their eyes to be teary after laser eye surgery. These symptoms usually subside within about six hours. For this reason, it's a good idea to take a nap following the procedure. Doing so will help you get through the most uncomfortable part of the healing process while experiencing minimal discomfort.

Postoperative Care

Plan to allow the rest of the day for rest and recovery. Most LASIK patients state they took a nap upon returning home

Over the course of the next few days, your vision should stabilize and continue improving. You may notice that your vision still appears somewhat smoky, as though you are trying to look through a smoke-filled room. In rare cases, it could take several weeks or longer for your vision to improve. Most people find their vision improves immediately after laser eye surgery, although the drops used in your eyes may temporarily cause blurriness.

It is a good idea to refrain from any form of strenuous exercise for at least a week after your treatment. This is because strenuous activity could result in trauma to the eye and affect the healing process. You should avoid the use of cosmetics for a minimum of one week following your procedure. You will also need to avoid swimming for up to two weeks following your surgery.

Expect to return to see your surgeon the day after your procedure. During this initial checkup, your surgeon will test your visual progress to make sure it's steady.

As is the case with any type of surgery, you should always follow our postoperative instructions and take any medication your surgeon prescribes as indicated. It's also important to avoid rubbing your eyes.

Follow-up visits will be scheduled approximately one week, one month, three months, six months, and one year after your laser vision correction procedure.

Most people experience only minimal discomfort after their procedure and are quite happy with the results of their laser eye surgery. If you have any concerns or questions, contact your LASIK surgeon right away.

Warning signs of complications include the following:

- Pain
- Decrease in visual acuity
- Redness in and around the eye
- Flashing lights
- Floaters

If you experience any of these symptoms, you should contact your surgeon immediately. Do not wait to see if the symptoms will improve.

COMMONLY ASKED QUESTIONS ABOUT LASER EYE SURGERY AND THE RECOVERY PROCESS

Will I Need to Use Eye Drops?

Yes. Your surgeon will provide instructions on how to use the correct dosage of drops. These drops are extremely important, as they promote the healing process.

Will I Be Able to Work the Day Following My Surgery?

Yes, but only if your surgeon says that your vision is stable enough. Whether you are able to work or not may also depend on the type of work you perform.

What Should I Do on the Day Leading Up to My Procedure?

You may do anything you like on the day before your procedure, as there is no anesthesia required for the procedure. There are no food or beverage restrictions.

Can I Go to the Gym after My Surgery?

It is best if you avoid any type of strenuous activity for at least seven days after your procedure. If you need to do anything that would cause you to sweat, please wear a sweatband to prevent perspiration from getting into your eyes.

Are There Any Restrictions Regarding Lifting or Bending?

No, there are no restrictions beyond avoiding any activity that might cause trauma to the eye or interfere with the healing process.

What Will I Be Able to Do Immediately After Surgery?

Your surgeon will advise that all LASIK patients go home and rest. Try to nap if you can. This will help promote the healing process on the first day. Taking a nap will help resolve most of the initial irritation you might experience following your procedure.

Can I Get in a Hot Tub or Go Swimming?

You should avoid getting any water in your eyes for at least two weeks after your surgery. Chlorinated water can increase the risk of infection and inflammation. You may shower, but you should try not to get water in your eyes. Also, try to avoid getting any soap or shampoo in your eyes for at least a week after the surgery.

Can I Wear Cosmetics?

On the day of surgery, you should not wear any makeup or perfume. You should not wear eye makeup for at least five days following your surgery. This includes mascara, eyeliner, or eyeshadow. When you do resume wearing cosmetics, use new eye makeup.

Can I Use Eye Creams after My Procedure?

You should not apply eye creams on the day of the procedure and for up to one week after the surgery. Applying lotions or creams to the eye area can put too much pressure on the eye and increase the risk of getting contaminants in the eye. If this happens, it could increase the risk of pain, inflammation, and infection.

What If My Work Environment Is Dusty?

You should always wear protective eyewear anytime you are in a situation in which there is a risk of getting something in your eyes. Also, you should wear UV-protective sunglasses when you are outdoors. You should try to avoid smoke, dust, or work in the yard for the first week following your procedure.

Will I Be Able to Drive Immediately after My Surgery?

No, you will not be able to drive immediately after your procedure. You will need to have someone drive you the day of the surgery. Your surgeon might prescribe a mild sedative to help you relax, which means it is recommended that you do not drive. However, most LASIK patients can drive immediately after their one-day postoperative appointment.

Will I Experience Any Pain or Discomfort?

Almost all patients experience some level of tearing, burning, and light sensitivity following laser eye surgery. The level of discomfort you may experience might range from hardly noticeable to quite irritating. This may depend on how your eyes respond and the type of technology that is used in your surgery. Discomfort usually dissipates within two to four hours. Your surgeon will advise you to take a nap after the return home. In most cases, patients wake up without noticing much discomfort. You may feel as though there is something in your eye. It's a sensation similar to having a lash in your eye. Although this can be bothersome, it is extremely important that you do not rub your eyes. Doing so could dislodge the corneal flap.

Will My Eyes Be Red Following the Procedure?

Some patients experience some redness following laser eye surgery. It is quite normal to have some dark red spots that are noticeable on the whites of the eyes. These spots may remain visible for several days following your procedure, as they are similar to bruising. In some cases, it could take several weeks for the spots to go away completely.

How Long Will I Need to Continue Using Artificial Tears and Prescription Eye Drops?

Ocular dryness is one postoperative side effect. Approximately half of all LASIK patients experience dryness following their surgery. This symptom usually lasts for only a few days following the procedure. Your surgeon should provide you with artificial tears to help minimize any discomfort you might experience. Along with using artificial tears, you may also be prescribed prescription eye drops to prevent infection and inflammation. These drops should be used as prescribed.

What Should I Expect from Follow-up Appointments?

On the day after your procedure, you will need to return to your surgeon's office for your first postoperative appointment. At this time, your surgeon will check your vision and verify that your corneas are healing as they should. You will have the chance to discuss any symptoms or discomfort you may be experiencing at this time. Future appointments will be scheduled and will occur at one month, three months, and six months postoperatively.

Will I Need to Wear Eye Shields at Night?

Your eyes will be fragile during the recovery process. It's a good idea to wear eye shields while you sleep. This helps promote the healing process and prevent you from rubbing your eyes. It is also a good idea to continue wearing the eye shields for the first five nights following your procedure. If you have children or pets sleep with you, it is important to wear the shields for up to two weeks following your procedure.

Will My Vision Be Hazy or Blurry after My Surgery?

While you should be able to see reasonably well the day after your surgery, you may notice that your vision is hazy or blurry for up to two weeks. The higher your original prescription, the longer it may take for your vision to clear during the recovery process.

Will My Vision Fluctuate?

Do not be concerned or surprised if you notice that your vision fluctuates somewhat following your procedure. Your surgeon will tell you what you should expect for your specific situation. Your reshaped corneas will need time to stabilize before your vision can stabilize. For this reason, you may experience some symptoms such as halos, glare, and difficulty driving at night during the first few days or even weeks after your surgery. In some cases, this could last for months. It is important that you always discuss any symptoms you are experiencing with your surgeon. If you believe your symptoms are abnormal or are lasting longer than they should, contact your surgeon immediately. Even if your vision is blurry, you should not resume wearing contact lenses unless you have received the go-ahead from your surgeon to do so.

What If My Vision Continues to Fluctuate or I Continue Experiencing Symptoms?

Haloes, glare, and difficulty driving at night, along with other visual symptoms, may continue while vision stabilizes. If further enhancement or correction is necessary, you will need to wait until your eye measurements have remained consistent for at least two consecutive office visits with at least three months between visits before your surgeon can perform another correction or enhancement.

DIFFERENCES IN RECOVERY BETWEEN PRK AND LASIK

Your recovery process may vary based on the type of procedure you have. There is no need to create a flap on the surface of the cornea in PRK. Consequently, there are some differences in the recovery period between PRK versus LASIK. In LASIK, the recovery period is usually much faster, allowing patients to return to work the following day. PRK, by comparison, usually requires a longer healing time. This is because a larger section of the front of the cornea, the epithelial layer, must be replaced compared to the relatively small section surrounding the flap that needs to heal in LASIK.

HOW TO ASSESS YOUR VISUAL SATISFACTION FOLLOWING YOUR FIRST PROCEDURE

A number of factors may affect your satisfaction following your first laser vision surgery.

- Whether you are far-sighted, near-sighted, or have an astigmatism
- The health and characteristics of your corneas
- The severity of your refractive error
- The strength of your prescription
- Your age
- Whether or not you are at risk for dry eyes
- Your own personal expectations

While laser eye surgery can correct high degrees of farsightedness, nearsightedness, and astigmatism, the best candidates for a good outcome are ones who agree in advance with the surgeon with the preferred postoperative results. Some people believe 20/20 vision is perfect vision, but it is not nearly as useful as being happy with your vision. For instance, younger patients with mild myopia may want a long period of contact lens-free vision while middle age patients might be very happy with the results of LASIK only lasting until cataracts begin to form.

As mentioned in Chapter 2, it is important to consider the phrase, "Is 20/20 Vision Good?®."

Your own personal expectations prior to your first procedure can also play an important role in how satisfied you are with your results. Keep in mind that the goal of this procedure is to decrease your dependence on contact lenses and glasses while helping you to see reasonably well without the need for corrective lenses. Every person is unique, so results will vary.

WHAT IS AN ENHANCEMENT?

An enhancement is a follow-up procedure that is performed in situations in which the outcome of the first laser vision surgery proved to be unsatisfactory or when your vision changes over time. Continual improvements in laser vision procedures and technology mean that re-treatments are only rarely necessary in order to enhance visual acuity.

Many studies have shown that the rate of enhancements has actually declined over the past several years. Even so, it should be understood that not everyone will be able to achieve crystal-clear vision with their first procedure. Every individual is unique, and numerous variables can affect the outcome of your procedure.

HOW DOES THE ENHANCEMENT DIFFER FROM THE FIRST PROCEDURE?

In most instances, an enhancement procedure is faster and simpler. This is because it is not necessary to lift the corneal flap, which is necessary in the initial procedure. A second procedure, or enhancement, is also identical to the first procedure. The only real difference is that instead of using a laser or microkeratome to create a corneal flap, the surgeon will use specialized tools to lift the flap that was created during your initial procedure. It only takes a minute or two to lift the flap, and it is completely painless. Your surgeon will use an excimer laser to reshape your cornea in the second procedure. In most cases, only minimal resculpting of the cornea is needed. As a result, the procedure is quite fast.

Usually, it is only necessary to perform a small amount of corneal reshaping for an enhancement. In most cases, all it takes is a single enhancement procedure to achieve desired results. While one enhancement is usually all that is necessary to restore a patient's vision to an acceptable level, more than one enhancement may be necessary in complex cases.

It should be understood that if you need a re-treatment, this does not mean that you have problematic eyes or that the surgeon lacks skill. This is simply something that cannot always be predicted prior to the first procedure. One of the reasons it can be difficult to predict whether an enhancement may be needed is the fact that the eye is 100 percent organic tissue. That being said, most enhancement surgeries are quite successful and can take your vision from quite good to excellent.

Following a consultation with your surgeon, you may decide that you do not want to undergo an enhancement. This could be the case if your vision is significantly improved and if you only notice slight problems in demanding light conditions. In such situations, you might be quite happy to wear glasses. This is entirely a personal choice.

After your enhancement procedure, you will need to follow the same postoperative instructions as during your first procedure. You should follow those instructions precisely to reduce the risk of infection and other complications.

OTHER ENHANCEMENT OPTIONS

LASIK enhancement procedures can be performed to improve vision following refractive surgeries other than LASIK, including refractive lens exchange and Intra Ocular Lens (IOL) implantation. In some instances, it may be necessary to perform a procedure other than LASIK for a patient's enhancement. For instance, PRK may be preferred over LASIK for an enhancement for a variety of reasons. PRK is sometimes preferred, as it offers a lower risk of surface cells growing under the flap. This is called epithelial growth. Enhancements can also be performed many years after the original procedure was performed. Both PRK and LASIK enhancements can also be performed following cataract surgery in order to eliminate any residual refractive errors that remain and sharpen the patient's vision.

If you have had any type of laser eye surgery in the past and believe that your vision is not as sharp as it should be, contact your LASIK surgeon's office to ask about an evaluation for a possible enhancement.

CHAPTER 5
CHOOSING A LASIK SURGEON

"It's the archer, not the arrow."

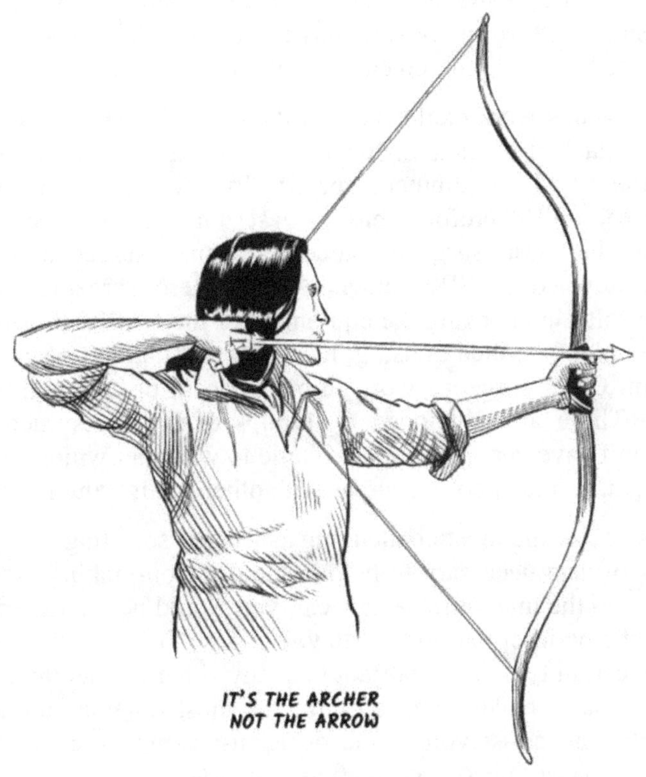

Once you have made the decision to have laser vision correction surgery, you're likely to feel excited about the opportunity to improve your vision as well as your overall quality of life. Before you take the step of actually having laser vision surgery, however, there is one final decision that needs to be made, and that is the decision of choosing the right laser vision surgeon for you.

The process of selecting a surgeon to perform your procedure can be somewhat confusing and challenging. One of the reasons for this is that few patients have ever actually shopped around for such a surgeon.

Your vision is important, and selecting a LASIK surgeon is a very crucial decision. You need a surgeon who is well trained, highly recommended by patients as well as doctors, and who has extensive experience. With so many surgeons from which to choose, it can be difficult to know whom you can trust with your eyesight.

Many surgeons work exclusively in their own LASIK center, which is often attached to their medical practice. This means the surgeon chose the LASIK equipment specifically for their own taste and preference, and therefore, has a vast amount of experience in creating the best surgical outcome. Some surgeons work in corporate-owned LASIK centers. While these surgeons typically have no roles in choosing the equipment or the LASIK process, they are often highly skilled at using the equipment that has been selected for them. Other surgeons work in open-access or community-based centers. These are developed by groups of LASIK surgeons who often don't have enough patient volume to warrant owning their own equipment, so they pool resources with other small-volume surgeons.

Perhaps one of the most challenging aspects of selecting a surgeon is the lack of data necessary to help in the decision-making process. If you were in the market for a new car, you would be inundated with a wealth of new information to help you choose the right vehicle. Your eyes are certainly more important than any vehicle. Therefore, it only makes sense to make sure you have the most reliable and accurate information to assist you in the decision-making process. When it comes to laser vision correction, complication rates, outcome statistics, and pricing information should all be considered.

UNDERSTANDING COMPLICATION RATES

It should be understood that even the best screened patients receiving care under the most experienced and skilled surgeons can sometimes experience complications during laser vision surgery. During the procedure itself, the malfunction of a device or other type of error could lead to damage to the eye or the need to discontinue the procedure.

After surgery, other types of complication rates may arise. Such complications may include inflammation, migration of the flap, and infection. These complications may require another procedure to be performed or additional treatment. It should also be understood that even with advanced therapy and treatment, some complications may result in vision loss.

If you are thinking about having LASIK performed and you are concerned that something might go wrong during your procedure, it is important to know that it is actually quite rare for complications to occur that would result in significant or permanent loss of vision. Furthermore, many complications can actually be resolved through an enhancement or retreatment. With that said, it should also be understood that complications can indeed occur. Consequently, you should carefully consider the risks associated with refractive surgery and the best way to minimize those risks.

Choosing the right surgeon is the most important step you can take to reduce any risks associated with laser vision correction surgery. A reputable, experienced surgeon will ensure you are a good candidate for the procedure. Should any problem occur during or after the surgery, an experienced and reputable surgeon will work with you closely to resolve those complications.

EXACTLY HOW COMMON ARE LASIK COMPLICATIONS?

Over the course of the past several years, public confidence in laser vision correction surgery has increased due to the success rate involving millions of successful procedures across the country. Due to the introduction of increasingly sophisticated technology used in laser vision correction procedures, the outcomes for most LASIK procedures are quite favorable.

The use of refractive surgery has even been adopted by the military in an effort to decrease the reliance of troops on eyeglasses and contact lenses.

HOW LASIK COMPLICATIONS DEVELOP

Serious complication rates can be held to less than 1 percent when surgical candidates are carefully screened. Prospective patients could be eliminated if they have certain medical conditions that might affect how well their eyes heal following the procedure. For this reason, it's important to discuss any health conditions that could affect your candidacy during your consultation.

As you may recall, large pupil sizes could also be considered risk factors for laser vision correction surgery complications. This is because in dark conditions pupils could expand beyond the area that was treated. If you have any concerns about this, it's important to discuss them with your surgeon.

Although the vast majority of outcomes for LASIK surgery are favorable, there is still a small percentage of people who experience continuing vision problems following their procedure. It should be noted that no surgical procedure is ever completely without risks.

Some patients with excellent vision may still experience side effects. For example, it is possible that a patient might have excellent visual acuity and then experience halos or glare around lights at night after having the procedure.

When complications do arise, they are often related to the hinged flap that is created in the cornea of the eye. This flap is lifted before reshaping the cornea with the use of a laser. The flap is then replaced so that it can form a natural bandage.

In the event the flap is not created properly, it is possible it might not adhere correctly to the surface of the eye. In some instances, the flap might be cut too thickly or thinly. Once the flap is put back into place on the surface of the eye, it might begin wrinkling. Such flap complications can result in an eye surface that is irregularly shaped.

The American Journal of Ophthalmology reports that flap complications occur between 0.3 percent and 5.7 percent of LASIK procedures. Higher rates of flap complications can be attributed to inexperienced surgeons. Keep in mind that you can boost your chances of avoiding LASIK risks by choosing a surgeon who is reputable and experienced.

TYPES OF LASIK COMPLICATIONS

Some of the most common problems related to LASIK flap complications include:

Vision Changes

You should be aware that if you have LASIK performed while you are in your 20s or 30s, it is likely your vision will change as you grow older. This is completely unrelated to your laser vision correction surgery. Instead, it is the result of normal aging, which includes a loss of focusing ability. This is known as presbyopia. Due to this, most patients who have had LASIK will need reading glasses at some point after the age of 40.

Under the care of an experienced surgeon, carefully screened candidates with a clear understanding of the risks and with reasonable expectations are most likely to be satisfied with the results of their procedure.

Irregular Astigmatism

A less-than-smooth corneal surface can result in irregular astigmatism. This complication can also occur from laser correction that is not centered in the correct position on the eye. Associated symptoms include double vision, or what is sometimes referred to as ghost vision. In such situations, the eye may need an enhancement or retreatment.

Diffuse Lamellar Keratitis

Also known as DLK, this complication is sometimes referred to as “Sands of the Sahara.” It is an inflammation that develops under the flap following LASIK surgery. This complication can lead to scarring of the cornea. Without prompt treatment, permanent vision loss can occur. Proper treatment includes topical steroids and antibiotics. In some cases, it may be necessary to remove inflammatory cells and have the flap relifted and rinsed to prevent tissue damage.

Ectasia

Post-LASIK ectasia is a condition in which the cornea begins to bulge forward at some time after the procedure. It may occur when a flap is cut too deeply or when too much of the tissue is removed. In some cases, ectasia may occur when the cornea is initially weakened. The resulting distorted vision usually cannot be corrected with the use of a laser enhancement. Instead, the surgeon may prescribe corneal implants or rigid contact lenses in order to keep the cornea held in place. Among the best ways to avoid this complication is for prospective patients to be examined prior to the procedure for certain risk factors. Among those risk factors are low residual stromal bed thickness, high myopia, and low preoperative corneal thickness.

Dry Eye

Approximately half of all patients who undergo LASIK report experiencing problems with dry eye during the first six months following their procedure. Such complaints are often associated with reduced sensitivity of the surface of the eye following the surgery. Patients experiencing problems with this complication can try temporary remedies such as prescription dry eye medication or artificial tears. Approximately six months to one year after the procedure, most patients find that such complaints disappear after the eye has completely healed.

Significant Undercorrection, Regression, or Overcorrection

An undercorrection or overcorrection of your vision means that you might experience slightly blurry vision due to residual nearsightedness, astigmatism, or farsightedness. Regression occurs when your vision is optimal at first after your procedure, but then begins deteriorating over time. This could be due to the return of some nearsightedness. Such problems can typically be corrected with a retreatment.

Eye Irritation or Infection

In some rare cases, patients may develop an eye inflammation, infection, or irritation that requires treatment. This type of infection can be potentially serious. Most cases of eye infections occurring during LASIK result from the native bacteria that can be found on the eyelids, edges of the lids, cornea, connective tissue, and tear canals. Pseudomonas and streptococci are the two most common bacteria resulting in eye infections following LASIK. Additionally, atypical mycobacteria and certain fungi may also be dominant in late-appearing infections. At times, certain viruses, such as enterovirus and herpes simplex, can result in post-LASIK infections.

Other sources of contamination that could result in an infection during a LASIK procedure include any sponges or instruments used during the surgery, ocular flora, airborne contaminants, and the hands of the surgeon and staff. For this reason, it is vital that patients choose a surgical center that is vigilant about cleanliness.

Patients with a post-procedure infection typically experience such symptoms as pain and loss of vision. Other possible symptoms may include haze, redness, increased sensitivity to glare, reduced best-corrected vision, irritation, and watery eyes.

When an infection is diagnosed following LASIK, it is crucial that the bacteria responsible for causing the infection be identified. This is because the antibiotic therapy used must target the bacteria as quickly as possible in order to yield the best results and ensure complete recovery. Delayed treatment could result in the need for additional surgery as well as complications, such as ulcers or abscesses within the eye. In the early stages of an infection, high-dose antibiotics are typically prescribed. Late-appearing or diagnosed infections may need to be treated with intravenous medications.

Mild cases of infection may be treated with the use of anti-inflammatory eye drops. In some cases, infection may progress to the point that the flap begins to melt. In severe cases, a particular type of intraocular infection known as endophthalmitis may occur resulting in dense scarring, visual impairment, and possible blindness. Depending on the severity of the infection, corneal transplantation may be required. Due to the fact that the flap never fully heals, patients who develop an eye infection following LASIK may be at risk for developing eye infections for the rest of their lives.

Eye infections typically occur within the first nine days following LASIK. In rare instances, such infections may manifest at a later time, typically between two to eight weeks following the procedure.

Risk factors that could increase the possibility of developing an infection include contamination during surgery, excessive surgical manipulation, use of local steroids, and rubbing one's eyes after LASIK. Patients with chronic herpes simplex, autoimmune disorders, and atopic eczema may also be at an increased risk for developing infection.

The best way to prevent or reduce the risk of an eye infection following LASIK is to use anti-infective eye drops. Additional measures should also be to minimize the chances of developing a late-appearing infection. Among those steps include choosing a qualified and experienced surgeon who will reduce the risk of infection during the procedure itself. Therefore, it's important to select a surgeon who will provide you with the proper diagnosis and recommend the treatment that is best suited for your particular situation.

Protective glasses should also be worn following the surgery to protect against rubbing the treated eye or eyes during the first 24 hours following the procedure, especially while you are sleeping.

If you do notice any redness, irritation, or pain in the treated eye following your procedure, it is vital that you follow up with your doctor as quickly as possible. This should be done regardless of whether your procedure was performed a few days ago, a few weeks ago, or a few months ago. If you experience any issues at all, you should follow up with your surgeon immediately. No surgery, even LASIK, is without risks and possible complications. Fortunately, the chances of developing an eye infection or other complication can be reduced.

Epithelial Growth

Although rare, epithelial growth is a possible complication of LASIK surgery. The incidence of epithelial growth following LASIK is about 1 percent following primary LASIK and less than 2 percent after enhancement procedures. Epithelial growth refers to the presence of corneal epithelium in an area where it should not be. Following LASIK, epithelial growth may take place between the stromal bed and the flap.

There are two ways that corneal epithelial growth can take place. One way is a loss of contact inhibition and another is during the microkeratome pass. When epithelial cells come into contact with the epithelium, they cease to grow. This is what is known as contact inhibition. Without contact inhibition, epithelial cells will begin growing in order to fill that space. In rare instances, when a buttonhole flap has developed in the flap, epithelial cells will actually make their way through the buttonhole and then enter the interface between the stromal bed and the flap.

Risk factors for epithelial growth include those patients with recurrent corneal erosion and those with corneal epithelial basement membrane dystrophy. Other possible risk factors include older patients, patients with diabetes mellitus, and patients who have had corneal surgery in the past as well as those who have had epithelial growth in the other eye. The best way to avoid epithelial growth is for patients to be screened very carefully. This is why it is critical to seek out a surgeon who will take the time to screen you to determine whether you are a good candidate for LASIK. Patients who have certain risk factor may have better results and be less likely to develop epithelial growth while undergoing PRK than LASIK.

It should be understood that there are also certain risk factors related to the surgery as well. These risk factors include partial flaps and buttonholes. Any time it is necessary to relift a flap while performing an enhancement procedure, the risk for epithelial growth increases.

FACTORS TO CONSIDER

In choosing a laser vision surgeon, it's important to take myriad factors into consideration. Below, we explore those factors to assist you in making an educated decision regarding your best choice for a LASIK surgeon.

Reputation

Among the most important factors to take into consideration when choosing a LASIK surgeon is the reputation of the surgeon. Keep in mind that while it is important to consider the opinion of the local community regarding the surgeon's reputation, ask for references and read online reviews. If there are any bad online reviews, ask the surgeon or surgical coordinator for an explanation of those particular situations.

Licensing, Training, Accreditation, and Certification

In the process of choosing a laser vision surgeon, it's important to make certain the surgeon you choose has advanced training in the proper field. Along with advanced training in ophthalmology, he or she should specialize in refractive and corneal surgery.

A surgeon who has attained board certification by the American Board of Ophthalmology will have passed a rigorous two-part exam. This exam is designed to assess the surgeon's experience, knowledge, and skills. It should be noted that only a small part of the board exam actually covers laser vision correction. The vast majority of the test actually covers the treatment and diagnosis of medical eye disease. Even so, board certification is still considered the ideal standard for the competence of a surgeon.

LASIK laser vision correction is not a subspecialty of ophthalmology. Rather, surgeons receive training in LASIK at some point during their residency, fellowship, or clinical practice. Surgeons who received a fellowship from an accredited training program in Corneal External Diseases and Refractive Surgery will have the most LASIK training prior to practice. Surgeons who received LASIK training as part of an accredited ophthalmology residency program will have the second-highest level of LASIK training. For those in clinical practice who have not had LASIK training formally led by professors of medicine, there are week-long or even weekend LASIK training courses available.

State licensing boards can assist patients in validating the credentials of a surgeon. For instance, credentials can be checked through the National Practitioner Data Bank or physician directory websites or apps.

Experience

Research has shown that the more experienced a surgeon is, the lower complication rates tend to be. When searching for a surgeon to perform your LASIK procedure, it is important to find one who is experienced, but it's also vital to understand what the word experienced means.

The number of years a surgeon has in the field of laser vision correction as well as the number of procedures performed are both important considerations in choosing a LASIK surgeon. You certainly do not want to be one of a surgeon's first patients.

Remember that there are a few caveats to this. For instance, some surgeons will include cataract procedures in the number of procedures they have performed. So, patients should ask specifically about the number of laser vision correction procedures the surgeon has performed. Additionally, while it is important to consider the number of procedures the surgeon has performed, the sheer number of procedures performed can sometimes be a poor indicator of quality. For example, a surgeon in a high-volume center might easily perform thousands of procedures per year but have very little experience in terms of providing quality preoperative or postoperative care, as these duties are assigned to an optometrist.

Such a surgeon could quite possibly lack the skill and knowledge of a surgeon who has provided a comprehensive level of care to a fewer number of patients.

Surgeons who only practice in high-volume centers typically do not offer any other diagnosis or treatment of eye conditions and diseases and, as such, are a poor choice for a long-term eye doctor. Surgeons in high-volume LASIK centers typically only perform LASIK and then move on to the next patient.

Experience in the Type of LASIK Procedure You Are to Have Performed

As you may recall, there are many different types of LASIK procedures. Do not be fooled by surgical centers that seem to have a significant amount of experience based on the number of patients who have had procedures performed at their facility. Laser vision correction surgery isn't fast food, and the number of people served is not as relevant as you might think.

It certainly is important to choose a surgeon who has abundant overall experience. However, it's equally important to select a surgeon who has performed a number of procedures of the type that you are considering having performed. This will help to eliminate any problems that might arise from a surgeon who is still undergoing the learning curve with a new procedure.

In order to take advantage of consistency in results, it's best to select a surgeon who also performs that procedure on a routine basis. This will help ensure the surgeon is able to maintain their skills.

Even though it may seem impressive that a surgical center reports having served a large number of patients, keep in mind that this could also indicate an excessively high-volume strategy where surgeons may cut corners in order to serve as many patients as possible. Look for a surgeon with lots of options to care for your eye health and improve your vision; if the surgeon's only tool is an excimer laser, all this physician can do is perform LASIK.

Known Within the Community

It's generally a good idea to choose a LASIK surgeon who is well known within the local community. This will help you to avoid a surgeon who is here today and gone tomorrow. You want avoid a surgeon who simply hides behind a corporate name and instead choose one who has direct visibility within your local community.

Actually, many surgeons who work for corporate centers are assigned to perform surgery at many corporate center locations and sometimes even in different states. Remember, these surgeons only provide LASIK surgery, not preoperative or postoperative care. So, while it's easy for them to travel from center to center five days a week, it is virtually impossible for the patients to meet that surgeon in advance, ask questions, or even discuss follow-up issues that may arise. In some cases, a corporate location does not meet the projected profit expectations, so the location is closed. This can leave patients who have undergone surgery at that location in a bind.

Always take the time to choose a surgeon in a location you feel confident will still be there in a few years rather than one who comes and goes.

Advertising

Many LASIK centers advertise on radio, television, the internet, and social media. Some still advertise in newspapers. There is certainly nothing wrong with this, but be aware that some advertisements provide more information than others. Be wary about deals or advertising that simply seem too good to be true. Remember that if a deal seems too good to be true, it probably is. Take the time to do your research.

Some vision correction centers will try to attract new patients by claiming that their facility has an impressive number of years of combined experience together. Such centers may claim to have performed an incredibly large number of procedures. Take care not to be impressed by such claims, as many of the national LASIK chains include the combined numbers of all of their LASIK surgeons nationwide. Keep in mind that your procedure will not be performed by all of the surgeons in the center. Instead, your procedure will be performed by one surgeon. Consequently, it's important to ask about the number of procedures the surgeon who will be performing your surgery has performed. Furthermore, ask about that surgeon's safety record.

If possible, ask the surgeon to provide you with the names and contact information of former patients. This will give you the opportunity to ask questions about their own experience with the surgeon and, more importantly, with their post-LASIK vision result.

Be sure to ask if the patient is happy with their vision.

If a surgeon performs too many procedures, say more than 20 or 30 per week, the surgeon often develops the mindset of a LASIK-only surgical technician, rather than retaining the mindset of an ophthalmologist.

Ask the center about the types of vision correction surgery they offer. If the facility only provides one type of surgery, this could indicate that the center does not offer individualized treatment. This means that you could experience less-than-ideal results. To avoid such problems, it's important to look for a laser vision eye center that will provide customized procedures. The more laser vision correction surgery options your surgeon offers, the more likely it is that you will receive a unique treatment plan that will reflect your overall health, eye anatomy, visual needs, and personal preferences.

Professionalism

From the time you enter the facility, you should be greeted with complete professionalism. The demeanor of the staff can speak volumes. Look for a facility with a staff that takes the time to listen to your concerns and who are willing to take the time to answer your questions and address your concerns. Expect to meet your surgeon, and ask to see the LASIK suite. Be sure to watch the 360-degree online video tour of the LASIK center before you arrive so you can compare what you see online to your actual visit.

Patient Satisfaction

What kind of success rate does the facility have? Naturally, you will want to choose a facility with a low rate of complications, but it's also important to be cautious about choosing a facility that boasts a 100 percent success rate. Unless a facility with that kind of claim can back up such claims with objective data, be wary.

Online Reviews

LASIK patients typically want to tell others about their life after LASIK. You should be able to find hundreds of online reviews about your LASIK surgeon and your LASIK center. If you cannot easily find a significant number of online reviews, you should independently ask the LASIK counselor and the LASIK surgeon why there aren't substantial online reviews. Think about their answers. Do the answers make sense to you? If not, it should draw concern as to whether the surgeon and the facility are technologically up to date.

Enhancements

Are enhancements frequently necessary at the facility you are considering? Keep in mind that laser eye surgery outcomes will vary based on the outcomes of individual patients. Even with a successful procedure, an enhancement may be necessary. Furthermore, patients may require eyeglasses for activities such as driving or reading. Due to the natural aging process, farsighted patients may experience vision that deteriorates over time.

Commitment to Results

Does the LASIK center offer a long-term commitment to their results? Does the commitment include enhancements? Because every patient's case is unique, it's important to discuss your own expectations with your surgeon, and your LASIK coordinator prior to your procedure.

DO'S AND DON'TS WHEN CHOOSING A LASER VISION SURGEON

When choosing a surgeon to handle your LASIK procedure, it's important to be aware of a few important things you should do as well as a few you should not do:

- Do not base your decision simply on cost alone. While it is certainly understandable that most people are looking to be budget-conscious, remember that you will likely get what you pay for.
- Do not simply settle for the first doctor, vision eye center, or procedure that you research. The decision that you make today about your eyes and vision will have an impact on the rest of your life and the quality of your life.
- Do be cautious about eye centers that advertise package deals or promise your money back if you do not receive specific results. If it sounds too good to be true, it probably is. Therefore, you should do your own research on LASIK pricing.

- Do read any information provided to you about your chosen procedure.

WHAT TO BE AWARE OF WHEN SELECTING A LASIK SURGEON

Even though LASIK is outpatient surgery, it should be kept in mind that it is still surgery. As is the case with any surgery, there are some patients who are not good candidates for this procedure. For instance, if you have unrealistic expectations or if you have certain contraindications, then you might not be the best candidate for this surgery. Furthermore, there are risks associated with laser vision correction surgery that should be reviewed and discussed carefully so that you have the opportunity to make the right decision regarding whether this procedure is right for you. The best way to learn about this procedure, including its risks, is to consult a surgeon specializing in LASIK. A LASIK consultation will provide you with the best opportunity to ensure your expectations are met.

Referrals

A good place to search for a LASIK surgeon is to ask relatives, friends, and coworkers. Think of all of the people you trust who have had laser vision correction surgery performed in the past, and ask them about the surgeons they have used. Remember to ask not only about their results but also how they feel they were treated throughout their surgical experience. For instance, were they treated in a friendly and competent manner? Were they encouraged to ask questions? Did they feel as though they were treated in a personal manner, or whether they were treated like just another patient? Asking for a referral is a great place to begin your laser vision correction consultation process.

QUESTIONS TO ASK A LASIK SURGEON

After you have found a LASIK surgeon, it's important to ask a few important questions to ensure he or she is the right surgeon for your needs. The best way to do this is to schedule an appointment for a consultation. This is an important meeting that should not be taken lightly. It provides the ideal opportunity to meet with the surgeon who will perform your procedure. To take full advantage of your consultation, take the time to write down relevant questions and ask those questions during your consultation. Don't feel shy about asking questions. Obtaining answers to questions can help put you at ease prior to your procedure.

- How many procedures have you performed? (When you ask this question, be sure to specify LASIK and PRK correction procedures.)
- How long have you been performing refractive eye surgery?
- How many of the refractive procedures that you plan to use for me have you performed? (This is an important question to ask. Even when a surgeon has performed hundreds of surgeries, there are always new techniques and technologies. You do not want a surgeon who is a rookie on a new technique or procedure.)
- What is your complication rate?
- How does your complication rate compare to the national average?
- How do you handle complications when they arise?
- Has your vision surgery center ever experienced a problem with serious eye infections?
- What is your policy for follow-up in the event of a complication?
- Do you belong to any professional associations?
- Have you completed any research or fellowship training?
- Is your board certification and licensure current?
- Which lasers (brand and model number) do you use?
- What is the percent of candidates that you decline for refractive surgery? (The only wrong answer to this question is "none." When a surgeon properly screens patients, some patients will be turned away because they are not ideal candidates for refractive surgery. A commonly quoted

statistic is that caring ophthalmologists turn away 5 to 15 percent of those persons seeking a laser vision consultation)

- What percentage of your patients have had enhancement surgery?
- What should I expect my vision to be like during the first weeks after my procedure?
- Can I expect my vision to fluctuate following my surgery? (An honest answer to this is "yes.")
- How long is the healing period?
- Will you require me to stop wearing my glasses or contacts prior to the initial exam? If so, how long? (The best answers are "yes" and "for several weeks to provide proper calculations.")
- Do you plan to measure the thickness of my cornea before making a surgical recommendation? (The answer to this should always be "yes.")
- How often will you perform postoperative exams? (The proper timeline for this should be one day after your procedure, one week, one month, three months, and six months).
- Would my leisure activities, occupation, or hobbies have any effect on my candidacy for surgery? (The answer to this should be "yes.")
- Are there any reasons why I might not be considered a good candidate for refractive surgery? (The surgeon you choose should answer "yes" and provide more detail about who is a good candidate for LASIK.)

QUESTIONS TO ASK THE SURGICAL COUNSELOR AT THE LASIK CENTER

- Do you perform procedures at your own center, or do you travel to other facilities?

- What are your outcome statistics?
- How do your outcome statistics compare to the national average?
- Does your center charge extra if enhancements are necessary?
- If you do not charge extra for enhancements, what is the cutoff date for addressing problems following the initial procedure?
- Can you explain all of the costs related to a vision correction procedure at your facility?
- How new are your lasers?
- Do you have experience in wavefront technology? (This is an important question because wavefront technology provides the ability to measure and correct farsightedness, nearsightedness, and astigmatism.
- Can you provide patient testimonials?
- Have you ever had a malpractice claim? (While it is quite possible that even a quality surgeon might have a malpractice claim on his or her record, it's important to look for a surgeon who has not had a lot of such claims and none in the recent past.)

FINDING THE RIGHT PERSONAL TOUCH

Although you might hear of a great surgeon practicing in another area, it's usually best to find someone who is near your own area. In the event that you do have a rare complication, it will be more convenient if you do not have to travel a long distance for appointments and follow-up care.

As is the case with any healthcare professional, it's important to find a surgeon you trust. You need to feel that you can really trust the individual performing your laser eye surgery and that he or she has a personal interest in your care. If you feel you lack rapport with your surgeon, there is reason to be concerned.

If everything goes well, you likely will not need to see your surgeon frequently. If, however, you are not happy with the results of your procedure or if you experience any issues with healing that might require more attention, then you will certainly want a surgeon who is personally interested in your care and who will work to address your concerns.

The front desk is the first impression you receive when you enter a laser vision correction center, and it can likely provide you with a good indicator of what you can expect throughout your interaction with that facility. For instance, consider whether staff members seem indifferent or whether they are friendly. Does the facility seem disorganized or competent? Is the staff willing to take the time to answer your questions?

Will the facility perform a comprehensive evaluation? Leading LASIK surgeons always begin each patient's consultation by performing a complete evaluation. During this exam, the surgeon will look for refractive errors and various health conditions, including corneal thickness, that might disqualify the patient from being a good candidate for LASIK. As previously discussed, it's not uncommon for a prospective patient to be rejected for LASIK because he or she simply is not a good fit for the procedure. An experienced and reputable LASIK surgeon will not perform surgery unless he or she is convinced the patient will actually benefit from the procedure and the risk of complications is low.

Taking the time to evaluate the personal touch offered by a facility is an important step in finding the right surgeon.

CONSIDERING OTHER REFRACTIVE PROCEDURES

As previously mentioned, it's important to consider the versatility and competency of a surgeon in a variety of procedures. Just because a surgeon only offers one refractive procedure, that does not necessarily mean that procedure is the best procedure for you. It's important to choose a surgeon who is experienced and comfortable with performing a variety of procedures, including LASIK, PRK, and clear lens replacement, also known as refractive lens exchange (RLE). Also, the surgeon should offer the latest technology.

If the surgeon you choose has a comprehensive understanding of a variety of procedures, he or she will be able to assist you in choosing the best procedure for correcting your specific vision problems. If your surgeon only performs one type of LASIK laser vision correction, you should seek another evaluation.

WHY BARGAIN PRICES ARE NOT ALWAYS THE BEST CHOICE

In the process of searching for a laser vision surgeon, you may come across surgery centers that advertise LASIK at incredibly low prices. For instance, you might see LASIK advertised as low as just a few hundred dollars per eye. If you take the time to read the small print of such advertisements, however, you will often see that such pricing is dependent on the patient's refractive error. In most cases, only a small percentage of patients will actually qualify for such low pricing.

Be careful to avoid the bait-and-switch advertisements. With this strategy, patients get pulled in by being tempted by a cheap advertised rate only to find out later that they do not qualify for that rate or that the rate being charged is only for LASIK performed with older technology.

Generally speaking, bargain-priced laser vision surgery is a basic procedure using a microkeratome to create the flap. Furthermore, this type of low pricing typically does not include follow-up visits, preoperative exams, postoperative medications, or treatments.

In some cases, a bargain laser vision eye surgery center will use a mobile laser. This means that the excimer laser, or femtosecond laser, is actually transported to the surgery center on the day of the procedure and will then be transported to another surgery center the following day. Such frequent movement of the lasers could affect its calibration, which in turn could affect the consistency of the surgery outcomes they produce.

Low-priced laser vision eye surgery centers also often only correct mild nearsightedness. If you have astigmatism, farsightedness, or moderate to high degrees of nearsightedness, then the cost of your surgery may be much higher than the advertised priced.

You may recall that LASIK has been around since 1989. Laser technology and surgeon techniques continue to advance and improve. A less expensive LASIK center will likely use less expensive and therefore older technology. Another way discount LASIK centers keep costs low is by skimping on training for the surgeon and the LASIK staff.

You always get what you pay for. What you want when it comes to the health of your eyes is a qualified surgeon with a lot of experience. Surgeons with fewer qualifications and less experience are more likely to charge less expensive prices. Taking the time to ask how active your surgeon is in terms of keeping up with the latest technology is an important step in choosing the right surgeon.

Remember that laser vision correction surgery is just that: surgery. Qualified surgeons spend a number of years perfecting their skills and will naturally charge a price that reflects their skill and expertise. While a surgeon with less experience might charge a lower price, you should ask yourself whether you are willing to serve as a learning experiment to save money on the cost of a procedure that can affect your vision for the rest of your life.

Keep in mind that you only have one set of eyes. The risk associated with a low-cost procedure simply isn't worth it. Fortunately, there are options available to help you save on the cost of laser vision correction surgery to help make it more affordable without resorting to a low-quality provider.

CHAPTER 6

LASER EYE SURGERY PRICING AND FINANCING

In many ways, LASIK should be viewed as an investment in yourself. While many people think nothing of dropping quite a bit of money on a vacation, a new gadget, or a new toy, they are often hesitant about spending money on themselves. If in the past the price of LASIK has turned you off the idea of having it or you have found yourself wondering whether it is really worth the money, it's important to take a few things into consideration to put the cost of LASIK into perspective.

If you are like most people who are considering having LASIK, you have likely already spent quite a bit of money on vision correction. One factor to keep in mind when you are considering LASIK and comparing pricing is to compare the one-time cost of LASIK to the recurring costs of contact lenses or glasses. On average, the lifetime cost of contacts is around $27,900. The average lifetime cost of glasses is around $10,000. As a result, the average individual could easily spend $500 per year and still have to cope with the hassles of eyeglasses or contact lenses. Over a period of 10 years, an individual relying on glasses or contact lenses could spend $5,000. When you compare the recurring costs of glasses and contact lenses, LASIK is actually far less expensive.

If you are still wondering whether the cost of LASIK would be worth it, consider the following questions:

1. **How old are you now?** The younger you are now, the longer you will need eyeglasses or contact lenses if you opt to not have LASIK. The longer you need corrective eyewear, the more money you will spend over the course of your lifetime. If you opt to have LASIK now rather than later, you

can enjoy great vision without the need to rely on glasses or contacts for years to come. Keep in mind, of course, that LASIK does not halt the natural aging process. At some point everyone develops cataracts. For some people, having LASIK just a few years before cataract surgery is warranted represents a great quality of life improvement compared to wearing glasses or contacts. While LASIK might be medically useful to someone just a few years away from needing cataract surgery, it is a personal financial preference to continue with contact or glasses until the time for cataract surgery is right.

2. **Do you have insurance?** If you have insurance with a vision plan, that plan could help to defray some of the costs of your glasses or contacts, but it would not cover all of the expenses related to vision correction. You will still need to take into consideration the cost of what you pay for the insurance premiums. Furthermore, some vision policies will actually provide discounts for vision correction procedures, including LASIK. If you aren't sure what might be covered, it would be a good idea to check your policy.
3. **Do you prefer the latest lenses and/or frames?** Are you the type of person who wants to have the latest lenses or frames? If you have vision insurance, it's possible that your policy might not completely cover certain anti-glare or protective coatings. Also, your policy may cover only a certain number of glasses during one year. This means that if you upgrade frequently or if you break your glasses often, you may need to pay the cost of additional pairs of glasses out of your own pocket. Over time, this can be a considerable cost.
4. **What type of contact lenses do you wear?** If you wear contact lenses, the type of lenses you wear can have a significant impact on the amount of money you spend annually on vision correction. It's not uncommon for popular daily disposable contacts to run about $600 per year. Over a period of 10 years, that could add up to $6,000. Over 20 years, you're looking at more than twice the cost of laser

vision correction surgery. Furthermore, as you age, your prescription will likely become more complicated. This typically results in even more expensive eyewear. If you wear soft or hard lenses, the cost of drops, solutions, and cases that are necessary for keeping your lenses sanitary can add up quickly.

There are many options available today for paying for LASIK. It may even be possible to finance the cost of your procedure. If you are still hesitant about whether LASIK is an affordable option for you, take the time to do the math for the amount you are currently spending on vision correction and find out whether LASIK might be a more affordable investment in the long term for your vision goals.

FACTORS THAT AFFECT LASIK EYE SURGERY COST

A number of factors can affect the cost of LASIK eye surgery:

- The type of surgical instrument used to create the corneal flap
- The type of laser technology used
- The reputation, experience, and skill of the surgeon
- Whether retreatments are covered in the fee
- Whether postop medications are covered in the fee
- Whether follow-up visits are covered in the fee

UNDERSTANDING WHY THE COST OF LASIK VARIES

First, it should be understood that the surgeon you choose will affect the price you pay for laser vision correction surgery. Surgeons with more experience tend to charge more than surgeons with less experience. This is because more experienced surgeons bring more expertise to your surgery. Consequently, many people tend to feel more comfortable working with an experienced surgeon.

Also, the technology used by your surgeon can affect the price of your procedure. Bladeless LASIK involves the use of a second laser that is not used in bladed procedures. This can increase the price of your procedure. A bladeless procedure provides many benefits, including precision and an easier and faster recovery. If you choose to add certain customizations to your procedure, such as topography-guided technology, this can also affect the price you pay for your surgery.

Always consider what is included in the quoted price. Some surgeons will quote a price for only the surgery without factoring in any additional services you may want or require.

LASIK SURGERY PRICING METHODS

A large number of refractive surgeons quote a single price only for LASIK. A small number of surgeons will quote different prices based on the type of technology used. In some instances, surgeons may quote a price based on the degree of refractive error as well as the vision correction required to effectively treat the patient. Generally speaking, LASIK surgeons and LASIK centers who use the latest technology will charge a single price. This means that such technologies are not charged separately as extra fees.

QUESTIONS TO ASK ABOUT PROCEDURE PRICES

As discussed, the cost of LASIK surgery varies based on a number of factors. Therefore, it should not be surprising that many patients have the same questions about the cost of LASIK. Below, we will cover some of the most common questions regarding the cost of laser vision correction surgery.

What is included in the cost of LASIK?

This is one of the most common and important questions posed about the cost of laser vision correction surgery. The answer largely depends on your LASIK surgeon and how services are structured. As we have discussed, some surgeons will quote a single price that includes everything, while other surgeons will quote a base price and then extra for additional services, such as aftercare. For this reason, it is important to ask the LASIK counselor exactly what is included in the cost of their LASIK procedure. If you are not sure about something, don’t be afraid to ask.

Is the cost for LASIK per eye?

The cost of laser vision correction surgery is generally charged per eye. Although most patients do have the procedure performed on both eyes, there could be situations in which a patient might choose to have the procedure performed on one eye due to their individual vision correction needs.

What about guarantees?

A satisfaction guarantee provides patients with re-treatment under certain criteria. For instance, re-treatment may be performed for a specific period of time following the completion of your procedure. When considering using a specific surgeon, always ask if any satisfaction guarantees are included with the cost of your procedure. A satisfaction guarantee will provide you with peace of mind.

Will insurance cover my LASIK surgery?

Insurance companies usually consider laser eye surgery to be an elective procedure. This means it is not typically covered by health insurance policies. The reason that most insurance companies do not cover laser vision correction surgery is that it is not thought to be medically necessary. This is because vision can be corrected with the use of contact lenses and eyeglasses. As a result, most major medical plans do not include LASIK as a benefit. The only exception to this is if your job requires perfect vision.

Even so, under certain conditions your procedure may be covered. Therefore, it would certainly be worth it to ask whether the procedure might be covered by your insurance company. As previously mentioned, it you have a vision plan with your insurance, it's possible that this plan would provide a discount for your LASIK procedure, so be sure to check.

Keep in mind that even if your insurance does not cover LASIK, there may be many affordable ways that you can cover the cost of LASIK.

For example, many surgery centers do provide financing options that give you the opportunity to pay for the procedure over time. You could also take advantage of tax-friendly savings options, such as flexible spending accounts and health savings accounts. These types of accounts make it much easier to save for the cost of your surgery.

LASIK FINANCING OPTIONS

It's completely natural to have questions about how to pay for your laser vision correction surgery. Although LASIK can certainly provide a number of benefits and improve the quality of your life, it is an expense. Therefore, you may have questions about the best way to make LASIK affordable.

MAKING LASIK MORE AFFORDABLE

There are a number of ways that you can make LASIK more affordable. While many insurance companies do not cover LASIK, some vision and medical vision plans will provide a discount if the surgery is performed by certain surgeons.

FSA

A flexible spending account (FSA) can be used to help in paying for laser eye surgery. With this option, you can divert some of your pre-tax salary into an account that can be used to pay for out-of-pocket health care. Be sure to ask your employer about whether they provide this type of account.

HSA

Another option is a health savings account (HSA). In order to be eligible for this type of account, you need to be covered by a high-deductible health plan at your place of employment. With an HSA, you have the option to add tax-free contribution to your health savings account each pay period up to a specified limit. An HSA differs from an FSA in that any money you do not spend in your HSA at the end of the year will roll over, which allows you to use it the next year. Based on your budget, you could possibly save enough money to cover the full cost of your surgery by making contributions to your HSA over a period of a couple of years or more.

Other Options for Paying for LASIK

Many refractive surgeons will offer financing plans to assist patients in affording LASIK. If you are in the military, there may be options to consider that might be available to you free of charge. Whether or not you are eligible will usually depend partially on the nature of your job duties.

Taking the time to invest in finding the right laser vision eye surgeon is a decision that will pay off well in terms of improved vision for many years to come.

CHAPTER 7

LASIK RE-TREATMENTS AND COMPLICATIONS

In the previous chapter, we discussed re-treatments and enhancements and why those procedures might be necessary. In this chapter, we will go into more detail about enhancements as well as other types of procedures to help you make the most informed decision regarding your laser vision correction surgery.

WHY ENHANCEMENTS MIGHT BE NECESSARY

As discussed, re-treatments or enhancements are follow-up procedures performed after an initial LASIK procedure. These procedures are performed if there is a need to still treat residual issues. Some individuals who have already had a procedure performed with earlier technologies may experience vision problems at night that can be alleviated with newer technology, including a custom topography guided treatment. Studies have shown that wavefront or topography treatments can help reduce nighttime vision problems as well as contrast sensitivity problems.

Complications from refractive surgery can be divided into those that are ablation- or healing-related, which usually require additional laser treatment, and those that are surgically induced and can therefore be managed. Examples of surgical complications include epithelial growth, corneal flap displacement, diffuse lamellar keratitis, and corneal flap irregularities. Examples of ablation- and healing-related complications include irregular astigmatism, spherical aberrations, and topographical abnormalities.

Crossover can exist, given that numerous induced complications result in a loss of contrast sensitivity, severe night vision disturbances, and a loss of best-corrected vision. Although it has been possible to manage surgical complications for quite some time, with the development of wavefront technology, it is now possible to evaluate patients in a comprehensive manner and thus offer additional possible treatment options. Topographically guided solutions are appropriate for a vast majority of patients. It should be kept in mind, however, that it is simply not possible to predict which individuals might be the most suitable candidates and who will have the best chances for full success.

It is also important to recognize that even if you did not have any problems with your original procedure, there is still a possibility that you could experience certain complications with an enhancement or retreatment procedure. All surgeries carry some degree of risk.

ALTERNATIVES TO ENHANCEMENTS

Re-treatments are sometimes necessary to correct any induced or remaining myopia, astigmatism, or hyperopia. There are no guarantees that a repeat procedure will actually correct these problems, however. Alternative types of vision correction include contact lenses; eyeglasses; and other specialized laser surgeries, inlays, or implants.

DETERMINING ELIGIBILITY FOR ENHANCEMENTS

Several factors help determine eligibility for enhancements. A re-treatment can also be performed once the patient's vision has stabilized following the original procedure. For most patients, this takes between one and four months. The higher the correction involved in the original procedure, the longer it typically takes for the cornea to heal properly. During the first two years following the procedure, the corneal flap can typically be lifted rather easily. In some cases, it's possible to lift the flap even several years after the original procedure. The best time to perform a re-treatment is when the refraction has stabilized. The patient must have a sufficient amount of corneal tissue remaining under the flap for the procedure to be performed safely. The amount of corneal thickness is a critical factor to be taken into consideration when determining whether an enhancement can be performed.

RETREATMENT TECHNIQUES

The technique for performing a re-treatment is almost identical to the primary procedure. During an enhancement procedure, it is necessary to relift the flap and move it out of the way so that the laser can be applied to the corneal bed. This type of procedure is performed by lifting the original corneal flap and applying a laser to the corneal bed. This is done using a specialized tool that helps the surgeon lift the flap. Lifting the flap is generally painless and only takes a couple of minutes to perform. An excimer laser is used to reshape the cornea. In most cases, only a minimal amount of reshaping is necessary, so it only takes a few seconds to perform.

The flap is then replaced immediately after the laser application. In most cases the cornea naturally holds the flap in place using a suction action. To protect the surface of the cornea, if necessary, a soft contact lens may be applied as a type of bandage for the first day.

Following the procedure, patients receive the same postoperative instructions as before their first procedure. It is important to follow these instructions carefully to facilitate the best outcome and reduce the risk of infection. In most cases, only one retreatment is necessary, but in rare cases, more than one retreatment may be required.

UNDERSTANDING COMPLICATIONS

First, please understand that complications from LASIK are quite rare. LASIK is a commonly performed laser vision correction procedure, and by choosing an experienced LASIK surgeon, the chances of anything going wrong are quite low. If you are concerned about success rates for LASIK, you should ask your surgical coordinator about your surgeon's success rate rather than looking at generalized, national trends because, once you have committed to having LASIK, only your eyes and your surgical outcome matters.

The risks related to the original procedure can apply to enhancement procedures as well. Some complications and risks can be long-term in nature. In severe complications, repeated or more invasive corneal surgery may be required. Such surgeries might include corneal transplant.

POSTOPERATIVE COMPLICATIONS AND SIDE EFFECTS

Patients may experience discomfort, pain, or foreign body sensation early in the postoperative period. Other side effects may include blurred vision, bright lights, fluctuations in vision, tearing, or dry eyes. Discomfort tends to be most common during the first few hours following the procedure. Patients should be aware that persistent pain is not usual and could indicate displacement of the corneal flap, a disturbance within the epithelial layer, or a possible infection. In the event of persistent pain, it's important to notify your surgeon immediately.

Corneal infection following enhancement procedures is rare, but it can be serious and result in corneal scarring, which would necessitate a corneal transplant. Corneal inflammation also can result from healing reactions or medications.

Following refractive surgery, some individuals experience a halo, starburst, or glare effect around lights or in low light situations. These disturbances can make it difficult to see well in dim light or drive at night. It is theorized that the risk for such disturbances increases with patients with high degrees of correction or with large pupils. This is a temporary condition in most patients that dissipates with time or can be corrected by using eye drops or wearing glasses while driving at night. In some patients, such problems remain permanent. Re-treatment may reduce residual refractive problems or improve night glare, but such procedures are limited by the amount of corneal thickness that remains, patient sensitivity to night glare, treatment area, and corneal healing pattern.

In some cases, patients develop a degenerative corneal disease known as keratoconus. In severe cases, this condition must be treated with a corneal transplant. Mild cases can be corrected with the use of contact lenses or glasses.

Repeat LASIK procedures can also result in undercorrection or overcorrection. If your surgeon wants to perform repeated LASIK procedures on you, then you should fully understand why, and perhaps seek a second opinion. Risks are associated with the variability in how patients heal as well as numerous other issues. Such complications can result in the need for some patients to wear contact lenses or glasses or even have another procedure.

Patients may also heal differently between eyes. Such differences depend on corneal curvature, preoperative prescriptions, and variations in healing. A difference in refraction between eyes is known as anisometropia. This condition tends to be most severe when only one has been treated and may result in eyestrain, loss of depth perception, double vision, headaches, and a need to wear contact lenses. Both anisometropia and farsightedness may cause muscle balance problems to worsen, which can lead to the eye wandering more.

In some cases, the eyes may return to their original prescription. This usually depends on the healing pattern of the patient, the severity of the original prescription, and other factors. Further procedures may need to be performed once the eye has stabilized, assuming there is a sufficient amount of corneal thickness left.

COMPLICATIONS OF THE CORNEAL FLAP

Corneal perforation is the most severe type of corneal complication. This complication requires corneal sutures or stitches. In many cases, an intraocular lens implant will be required because the natural lens is damaged or lost. Corneal perforation could also result in infection and the need for a corneal transplant to be performed. While other risks do remain, the risk related to flap creation can be avoided when a retreatment is performed by lifting the original flap. Other possible risks include wrinkling or displacement of the flap and epithelial growth.

Complete or partial corneal flap displacement may take place during the first few days following the procedure or even weeks later after some kind of trauma. For this reason, it is important to protect the eye from any type of trauma. Patients should avoid rubbing the eyes after an enhancement procedure. Partial displacement of the corneal flap may cause corneal wrinkles or striae, which can cause blurred vision. In most cases, such striae can be treated, but in rare cases, treatment may not be possible. Complete displacement of the corneal flap requires immediate replacement. The risk of infection and epithelial growth is higher with complete flap displacement.

CORNEAL HEALING COMPLICATIONS

Corneal healing problems tend to be most common in patients who have corrected higher prescriptions. Such problems may affect the speed of the healing process as well as the smoothness of the cornea. This can result in corneal scarring and blurry vision. Corneal irregularities can also affect the crispness, sharpness, and quality of the final resulting vision. Corneal astigmatism and irregularities occur when corneal healing takes place in an irregular manner. While it is normal to expect corneal irregularities during the first few weeks following a repeat procedure, if they persist beyond six months they are abnormal in nature and usually permanent.

Irregular astigmatism from surgical complications and healing can cause a loss of best-corrected vision. Patients who experience this problem may not be able to read the last few lines on an eye chart even while wearing contact lenses or glasses.

Expectations

The overall goal of a re-treatment is to achieve the best possible visual result with the safest technique while significantly reducing the patient's need to depend on contacts or glasses. Patients may still need to wear reading glasses or glasses while driving at night. The degree of correction required will determine the initial accuracy of the procedure as well as the rate of recovery. Severe degrees of nearsightedness may necessitate multiple procedures. After the first procedure, even when additional surgeries are performed, patients may still have some remaining farsightedness, nearsightedness, or astigmatism.

Patients who have high refractive errors, astigmatism, and who are older than 40 are most likely to require enhancement following LASIK. A study published in *Ophthalmology* found that even three years after a primary LASIK procedure, the manual flap lift technique can still be quite successful. While older patients typically do quite well, the study found that the outcomes of older patients are not as predictable as the outcomes for younger patients. Patients with astigmatism and high refractive error are also more likely to require enhancements. This does not indicate a bad result, but it is important for patients to understand their situation and discuss their expected outcomes for their situation with their surgeons.

Both PRK and LASIK retreatments may also be performed following cataract surgery in order to sharpen vision and eliminate any residual refractive errors.

KERATOCONUS

Keratoconus is a type of progressive eye disease. In this disease, the cornea typically begins to thin and bulge out into a cone-like shape. As a result of the cone shape, light is deflected as it enters the eye, resulting in distorted vision. This condition may occur in both eyes or just one eye. It usually begins developing in an individual's teens or early 20s; however, a small number of reported cases have occurred after LASIK laser vision correction.

Treatment for Keratoconus

Mild forms of keratoconus can be treated with soft contact lenses or eyeglasses. This is a progressive disease; as such, when the cornea continues thinning and becomes more irregularly shaped, soft contact lenses and glasses may no longer provide sufficient vision correction. Treatments for this condition may include the following:

- Custom soft contact lenses
- Corneal cross-linking
- Hybrid contact lenses
- Gas permeable contact lenses
- Conductive keratoplasty
- Corneal transplant

CORNEAL CROSS-LINKING

This procedure, also sometimes called corneal CXL, works to strengthen a patient's corneal tissue to put a stop to the cornea's bulging as a result of keratoconus. This is a rare treatment option that combines the use of ultraviolet light with corneal immersion in riboflavin.

CONTACT LENS OPTIONS

Many types of contact lenses may be used to treat keratoconus. These are often customized and always highly specialized for the patient's condition. If you develop keratoconus, be sure to ask your eye doctor about all of the contact lens specialty options available to you.

CORNEAL TRANSPLANT

Corneal transplant is a surgical procedure where the damaged corneal tissue is replaced with healthy donor tissue. This is most often performed by an ophthalmologist who has completed extra training, called a fellowship, in cornea and external disease. While this might sound scary, the success rate for corneal transplant is extremely high and the procedure is performed on an outpatient basis.

CHAPTER 8

CATARACT AND REFLECTIVE LENS EXCHANGE (RLE) AND OTHER LASIK ALTERNATIVES

Although the development of cataracts can be a frightening prospect for most people as they grow older, it is important to understand that some possible treatment options, such as lens exchange, are available.

UNDERSTANDING HOW CATARACTS FORM

Cataracts form as clouding over the natural lens in the eye. The lens is located behind the pupil and the iris. In people over the age of 40, cataracts are the most common form of vision loss. They are also the primary cause of blindness. According to Prevent Blindness America, there are more cases of cataracts around the world than there are of diabetic retinopathy and macular degeneration combined. Cataracts are estimated to affect more than 22 million people over the age of 40 in the United States.

There are different types of cataracts. They include, but are not limited to the following types:

- **Subcapsular Cataract:** This type of cataract develops at the back of the lens. Individuals taking high doses of steroid medications and those with diabetes have a higher risk of developing this type of cataract.
- **Nuclear Sclerotic Cataract:** This type of cataract refers to the hardening of the center of the lens of the eye.
- **Cortical Cataract:** A cortical cataract features white opacities in the periphery of the lens that work their way outward in a spoke-like manner.

SYMPTOMS OF CATARACTS

Cataracts typically begin small and usually have no immediate effect on a person's vision. Someone with cataracts may notice slightly blurry vision at first. Blurred or hazy vision is the most common symptom of cataracts. Light from a lamp or the sun might seem too glaring or bright. While driving at night, you might notice that the glare from oncoming headlights is brighter than usual. Colors may not appear as bright as they did in the past. The symptoms you experience will be affected by the type of cataract you have. In the case of a nuclear cataract, you might actually experience a temporary improvement in your near vision. This is referred to as second sight. Sadly, this is only temporary, and as the cataract worsens, the improvement will disappear. On the other hand, subcapsular cataracts may not produce any symptoms until the cataract is well developed.

CAUSES OF CATARACTS

The lens inside the eye works like the lens of a camera. It focuses light onto the retina to produce clear vision. It is also responsible for adjusting the focus of the eye, which makes it possible to see things clearly. The lens of the eye is composed primarily of protein and water. The proteins in the lens are arranged in a very precise manner to keep the lens clear while allowing light to pass through. As a result of the aging process, some of the protein inside the lens may begin clumping together and begin to cloud. This is how a cataract first forms. Over time, the cloudiness may grow larger and cover more of the lens, which makes it more difficult to see. Although researchers are not certain why the lens changes as a result of the aging process, risk factors may include the following:

- Hypertension
- Ultraviolet radiation
- Diabetes
- Smoking
- Obesity

- Eye strain
- Eye inflammation or injury
- Statin medications
- Prolonged use of corticosteroid medications
- High myopia
- Hormone replacement therapy
- Significant consumption of alcohol
- Family history

It is also believed that cataracts may form as a result of oxidative changes that take place within the lens. Nutritional studies have shown that the consumption of fruits and vegetables high in antioxidants may help to prevent the development of certain types of cataracts.

PREVENTING CATARACTS

There is some debate as to whether it is possible to prevent the development of cataracts. Even so, some studies indicate that nutritional supplements may help reduce the risk of developing cataracts. Specifically, food sources that are high in Vitamin E may prove to be helpful. These food sources include almonds, sunflower seeds, and spinach. Foods that are high in zeaxanthin and lutein may also be beneficial. These food sources are green leafy vegetables, such as kale and spinach. Other research has found that foods containing omega-3 fatty acids and vitamin C may reduce the risk of cataracts.

WHEN TO CONSIDER CATARACT SURGERY

When the symptoms of cataracts first begin appearing, it may be possible to temporarily improve vision by using new eyeglasses. Surgery may need to be considered when cataracts have developed to the point that vision is seriously impaired. While poor vision is accepted as part of the natural aging process, it should be noted that cataract surgery is a relatively painless and simple approach to regaining vision.

Cataract surgery is a commonly performed procedure that can be quite effective at restoring vision. Each year, more than three million people undergo cataract surgery and approximately 90 percent of people who undergo this procedure are able to regain very good vision, falling somewhere between 20/20 and 20/40 vision.

WHAT TO EXPECT DURING CATARACT SURGERY

During the procedure, the clouded lens will be removed and, in most cases, replaced with a clear, plastic intra ocular lens (IOL). As a result of ever-advancing technology, new IOLs are being developed frequently to provide more benefit to patients. For instance, a presbyopia-correcting IOL makes it possible for patients to see at all distances. Other types of new IOLs include those that block ultraviolet light.

What Is CLE and RLE?

Clear lens extraction (CLE) is also known as refractive lens exchange (RLE) and presbyopic-correcting IOL exchange.

Types of IOLs

There are different types of IOLs:

- **Phakic IOLs**

  These implantable lenses avoid the need to remove corneal tissue. They are inserted into the eye directly in front of the natural lens.

- **Refractive Lens Exchange**

  This type of lens replaces the natural lens using an IOL with a different power in order to correct vision. RLE is sometimes a better option for patients with high hyperopia or presbyopia than phakic IOL refractive surgery, PRK, or LASIK. RLE can help reduce the need for bifocals or reading glasses by providing sharper focus and correcting refractive errors. The best candidates for this procedure are those who are not eligible for phakic IOL or LASIK because of their presbyopia or hyperopia. The procedure takes about 15 minutes per eye and is typically able to produce clear vision at all distances without contact lenses or glasses.

Lens replacement may also help correct myopia but is typically not recommended for patients who are eligible for phakic IOLs, PRK, or LASIK.

There are three types of IOLs that may be used to replace the natural lens of the eye. The type of lens that may be used is based on the health of the eyes and the patient's vision needs. These are the three types:

- **Monofocal Fixed-Focus IOLs**

  Monofocal lenses offer clear vision at a distance as well as intermediate and near ranges. It should be noted that these types of lenses do not produce clear vision for all three distances simultaneously.

- **Multifocal IOLs**

  This type of lens offers clear vision at multiple types of distances.

- **Accommodating IOLs**

  This type of lens enables the patient to focus at multiple distances by shifting the position of the lens within the eye.

There is no single lens that is a one-size-fits-all solution. Your surgeon will recommend the type of lens that is best for you based on your individual needs.

With RLE, the procedure is performed on an outpatient basis. Both eyes are not done at once and instead need to be done separately, about one week apart. Because numbing drops are placed in the eyes during the procedure, most patients usually do not experience any discomfort. Immediate vision improvement is typically reported following surgery. The initial recovery from RLE is about one week.

The final outcomes of RLE may take up to several weeks. During this time, patients may notice some visual disturbances, including halos, glare, blurry vision, and feeling a somewhat scratchy sensation in the eyes during the healing process. Patients are typically able to return to work and return to driving within one week of surgery. Most patients never even notice the presence of an IOL in their eye. Because the lens is actually inside the eye and is not positioned on the surface in the same way as a contact lens, others won't notice it either. These lenses are designed to last for the rest of a patient's life. Patients should be aware that there is a minimal risk of vision regression over time.

Presbyopia affects most people and becomes more noticeable sometime after the age of 40. This naturally-occurring age-related condition causes the natural lens of the eye to become firmer and therefore less flexible. As a result, patients are not able to focus on near objects. Non-surgical treatment options for presbyopia may include bifocals, reading glasses, or progressive lenses. Contact lenses for monovision may also be a treatment option. Refractive surgery, such as PRK, LASIK, and phakic IOLs are not able to directly address vision loss as a result of presbyopia. Although recent developments have been made available, not all patients are suitable candidates for procedures such as CK or monovision LASIK. RLE is often the best surgical option for individuals with moderate to severe hyperopia and presbyopia.

COMPARING RLE WITH LASIK

Although LASIK is still the most popular surgical option for the correction of hyperopia and myopia, patients with severe refractive errors or who have an abnormal cornea may benefit from a lens-based refractive surgery such as phakic IOL implantation or clear lens extraction.

Unlike PRK or LASIK, almost any degree of hyperopia can be corrected with refractive lens exchange. Furthermore, visual acuity is typically better after RLE than following PRK or LASIK in cases of moderate to high hyperopia. RLE is typically only performed on patients who are not suitable candidates for other types of vision correction surgery. Individuals with myopia may experience a higher risk of retinal detachment during RLE.

WHAT TO EXPECT FROM VISION FOLLOWING REFRACTIVE LENS EXCHANGE

Whether a patient will need contact lenses or eyeglasses following refractive lens exchange will depend on the type of lens that is used in the procedure. Monofocal IOLs are used frequently in both clear lens exchange as well as cataract surgery. This is because they provide excellent contrast sensitivity and vision while producing low incidences of vision disturbances, such as glare and halos. With that said, because monofocal IOLS are designed to focus only at a single distance, patients will likely require eyeglasses for close-up work, such as working at a computer or reading fine print.

A significant development in intraocular lens surgery is the FDA's approval of multifocal and accommodating IOLs, which provide vision at multiple distances and reduce or eliminate the need for glasses or contact lenses.

Most importantly, vision improvements from RLE often stay with you for life, as these advanced lens implants are engineered to adapt and offer you continuing visual enhancements as you age.

RISKS AND SIDE EFFECTS OF RLE

RLE is performed in much the same way as a cataract procedure. As a result, potential complications are approximately similar to cataract surgery. Because lens replacement surgery is a more invasive procedure than LASIK or other laser-based refractive surgeries, there does tend to be more risk. Even so, complications that would threaten a patient's vision are rare. Most complications associated with RLE can be treated quite well with medication. In some cases, an additional surgery may be necessary. Although RLE has been shown to be quite effective and safe, it should be understood that any type of surgery comes with some level of risk. The possible risks and complications related to RLE include the following:

- Dislocated IOL
- Retinal detachment (most common in people with extreme nearsightedness)
- Droopy eyelid

- Increased eye pressure
- Halos, glare, and blurry vision
- Bleeding or infection inside the eye

ADVANTAGES OF RLE

Despite the possible complications and risks of RLE, this procedure offers a number of advantages, including a very fast recovery. Also, there is an excellent predictability of outcome and superior quality of vision.

IMPLANTABLE COLLAMER LENSES

Since PRK and LASIK were introduced in the mid-1990s, they have successfully helped millions of people see better without the need for contact lenses or glasses. Laser eye technology has continued to progress since that time, making it possible for patients to enjoy more consistent results. Despite these advances, there are still many patients who are simply not good candidates for either LASIK or PRK. Patients who have extremely high prescriptions or those with irregularly shaped or thin corneas or severely dry eyes or even a combination of these factors may not be suitable candidates for PRK or LASIK, but they might be excellent candidates for ICL.

Losing, breaking, or misplacing one's eyeglasses is an annoyance for many people, but for individuals who are extremely nearsighted, the inability to wear glasses or contacts can mean not being able to see at all. For such individuals, implanted collamer (contact) lenses can be quite beneficial.

WHAT ARE IMPLANTABLE COLLAMER LENSES?

These lenses are implanted surgically in the eye in front of the eye's natural lens. They bend light rays onto the retina so that a clear image can be formed. Research has found that this procedure is just as safe as LASIK. This procedure is best suited for people who have moderate to severe myopia (nearsightedness). ICL has served as an alternative for many vision correction surgery patients for a number of years. It is sometimes an option for individuals with thin corneas who may not be suitable candidates for LASIK.

Among the benefits of this procedure is that it is not necessary to remove any corneal tissue. A small self-sealing incision is made. The lens is inserted through this incision. No stitches are required. Because the lens is inserted in front of the natural lens and behind the iris, observers cannot see it and patients cannot feel it. Vision is usually significantly improved immediately after the procedure. Over the next few days, vision tends to continue improving. As is the case with all surgeries, there is some degree of risk with this procedure. In order to reduce risk, it's important to select a surgeon with experience performing this procedure. Potential benefits and risks of this procedure should be discussed with the surgeon prior to the procedure to determine whether you are a good candidate for this procedure.

Why Choose ICL?

ICL may be a good option for people who are not good candidates to undergo LASIK, such as those who have corneas that are too thin or those who have a prescription that is too strong for laser vision correction. It should be noted that not all surgeons are experienced with performing this procedure, so it is important to find a surgeon who has experience in performing ICL. This procedure is often preferred because it offers a permanent way to correct one's vision as well as the possibility of the lenses being removed or adjusted when necessary.

What Happens during the Procedure

ICL is a relatively fast and painless procedure that is performed on an outpatient basis. No laser is required for this surgery. When necessary, it can be reversed by performing an additional procedure to remove the lens.

This procedure can be performed in less than half an hour. Prior to the procedure, a topical or local anesthetic will be used to numb the eye. If necessary, a mild sedative may be given. ICL is much like an intraocular lens implant surgery. The exception is that there is no need to remove a cataract prior to placing the lens. This makes it possible for the lens to be inserted without the need to remove the natural lens in the eye. An implantable contact lens is inserted and put into place in front of the natural lens instead.

Recovery for ICL

The recovery for ICL is somewhat similar to that of IOL surgery. It is necessary for patients to follow up with their ophthalmologist within 24 hours of their procedure. Eye drops along with a protective shield will need to be used in order to protect the eye during the healing period. Over-the-counter pain medications can be used to treat any minor pain following the procedure.

Patients are usually able to observe improved vision on the same day of their procedure. Optimal effects can typically be observed within one to seven days of the surgery. The total recovery period for ICL is generally short. Patients usually find that their eyes are healed completely within one to two months.

It may be necessary for patients to update their ICL prescriptions as they age. Some research indicates that most patients' prescriptions remain fairly constant, which eliminates the need to have the original lens replaced with a lens of a different strength.

ICL COMPARED WITH LASIK

ICL is quite similar to LASIK in many ways. For instance, both procedures involve the use of anesthetic eye drops. In some instances, a mild sedative may be used. Both procedures can be used to correct nearsightedness, although LASIK can also be used to correct farsightedness and astigmatism. Both procedures offer a short recovery period of only a few days. The vast majority of patients who have either surgery report being satisfied with their procedure results.

Who Is a Good Candidate for ICL?

Patients who have been told they are not good candidates for LASIK due to thin corneas or high refractive errors may be good candidates for ICL. The best candidates for this procedure are between the ages of 21 and 40 who have moderate to severe nearsightedness. Ideally, the patient should have healthy eyes and should not have had any previous eye surgeries. Patients who may not be good candidates for

LASIK, including those who have high degrees of nearsightedness or those with keratoconus, are often excellent candidates for ICL. The best way to determine whether a patient is a good candidate for this procedure is to have a comprehensive eye exam.

Patients should also have a stable prescription and should have realistic expectations regarding both the benefits and risks of ICL surgery as well as possible alternatives.

<u>Advantages of ICL</u>

Among the advantages of ICL is the fact that it can correct a wide range of nearsightedness without the need to damage or remove any corneal tissue, and because the lens does not change any structures within the eye permanently, it can be exchanged or even removed as necessary. The ICL can also be used even in patients with thin corneas, large pupils, or dry eyes. This procedure is also capable of providing predictable outcomes. Because the lens is constructed of collamer, it is quite biocompatible. There are no physical limitations following an ICL procedure. Most people find they are able to return to their normal daily activities not long after their procedure.

The ICL will not become dirty in the same way as a normal contact lens. There is no need for maintenance because the lens will remain clear, although it will be necessary for the patient to have an annual eye exam.

In the event there are vision changes, it is possible for the ICL to be replaced or removed. If necessary, eyeglasses and even contact lenses can be worn.

It is important to note that ICL cannot help presbyopia, which is caused by age-related vision loss. While ICL can provide near-normal vision, patients who experience normal distance vision may need to eventually use reading glasses for near work. This usually begins to take place once a patient reaches his or her 40s, regardless of whether they have had this procedure or not.

In the event the patient develops cataracts, it will be necessary to remove the ICL along with the cataract and implant a different type of lens.

CORNEAL INLAY

From the time an individual is born, the eye's natural lens begins hardening. As a result, it loses flexibility. This continues throughout life. Most people do not even notice this process until after they are in their 40s, when the inflexibility makes it difficult to focus on near objects. This loss of near vision, presbyopia, is natural but can be frustrating. Eventually, most people require reading glasses in order to see computer monitors and print clearly.

An inlay treatment can help improve near vision while giving patients freedom from reading glasses. The inlay is positioned in the clear tissue located at the front of the eye, the cornea. Thinner and smaller in size than a contact lens, the inlay is actually a type of mini-ring that features a small hole in the center. This pinhole is used to help focus light entering the eye, thus improving near vision while still maintaining distance vision.

Why Choose Inlays?

There are a number of reasons for choosing this treatment, including the fact that it can eliminate or reduce one's dependency on reading glasses. Additionally, there is little to no discomfort involved, and the procedure time is relatively quick. This procedure can also be performed on an outpatient basis, and patients can enjoy minimal downtime. Most people are able to resume their normal activities by the following day. There are no sutures necessary, and no corneal tissue is removed in the procedure. The inlays can be removed or replaced as necessary.

How the Inlay Works

The corneal inlay has been approved by the FDA for treatment in presbyopic patients between the ages of 45 and 60. It is usually implanted only in the non-dominant eye. The lens itself is smaller than a contact lenses and measures only 3.8 millimeters across. The small hole in the center of the lens has a 1.6 millimeter aperture. Instead of adding focusing power or changing the shape of the cornea, the inlay extends the patient's range of vision, providing long-term performance. It only takes about 15 minutes for the inlay to be implanted.

Who Is a Good Candidate for Inlays?

Patients who plan to have this procedure should be at least 45 years of age and have stable vision. There should be no history of eye disease. Patients should also have realistic expectations of the procedure, including the potential risks and complications.

Possible Risks and Complications of Inlays

As is the case with all surgeries, there are certain risks and complications related to this procedure. These risks and complications include the following:

- Reduced quality of vision
- Infection
- Night vision problems
- Halos or glare around lights
- Blurriness
- Fluctuating vision

Some complications of this procedure may be temporary, but other complications may require follow-up surgery to treat. Furthermore, some patients may find they still need to wear glasses in certain situations. In cases in which the inlays need to be removed, it may be possible for them to be replaced with a different lens. It should be understood that there is always a risk that one's vision will not return to where it was prior to the inlay procedure.

What to Expect from the Procedure

From beginning to end, the procedure usually takes less than 20 minutes. To ensure patient comfort, numbing drops are used throughout the entire procedure. Patients may observe a slight pressure as a small pocket is created with the use of a laser. This pocket is created in order to place the inlay in the cornea. It only takes a few seconds for this part of the procedure. Next, the inlay is placed in the pocket. Patients may notice their eye feeling scratchy or irritated once the numbing drops have worn off. There may also be some light sensitivity or excessive tearing. This is normal.

Medications may be prescribed to help patients manage these symptoms.

It should be noted that this procedure is a surgery and as such does require some healing. It is important for patients to follow the postoperative instructions provided to help speed along the healing process. The amount of vision improvement experienced typically varies among patients. Although some patients may notice an improvement in their vision within the first week, other patients may not notice any improvement until later. Most patients are able to resume their normal daily activities and even return to work by the next day or at least within 48 hours.

Patients should avoid the use of reading glasses and make sure they follow all other postoperative instructions, including the use of artificial tears in order to enhance the recovery process and near vision improvement. It's also important to keep all follow-up appointments.

It is normal to experience some vision fluctuations during the first three to six months following this procedure. This generally indicates that the brain is working to adapt to the patient's new vision. In most cases, the patient's vision will stabilize.

Now that you have a good understanding of some of the alternatives to LASIK that are currently available and the circumstances in which those procedures might be most suitable, you will be better able to make the most informed decision regarding which procedure might be best for your own situation. In the next chapter, we will discuss some of the most commonly asked questions about LASIK, including what to expect before, during, and after the procedure. We will also provide a glossary of terms to help you better understand what is involved in the many different types of laser vision correction procedures.

CHAPTER 9
COMMONLY ASKED QUESTIONS ABOUT LASIK

The decision to have LASIK surgery is certainly a big one. When you are considering having any type of surgical procedure, it's important to make sure you are well informed.

The following commonly asked questions are designed to help you find answers to your questions quickly and easily, ensuring you are able to make a well-informed decision about whether LASIK is the right procedure for you.

WHAT IS LASIK SURGERY?

LASIK surgery helps reduce or even eliminate the need for contacts or eyeglasses. An excimer laser is used to gently reshape the cornea in order to correct astigmatism, farsightedness, or nearsightedness.

Laser vision correction involves the use of a cool (nonthermal) beam of light to reshape the cornea, or surface of the eye, to improve vision. The laser works to remove microscopic bits of tissue to flatten the cornea in order to correct nearsightedness, smooth out irregularities in the cornea to treat astigmatism, or steepen the cornea to correct farsightedness. The goal of laser eye surgery is to change the shape of the cornea so that it works better at focusing images onto the retina, resulting in sharper vision.

IS LASIK THE RIGHT SURGERY FOR ME?

LASIK surgery offers a tremendous amount of potential to enjoy a life without the need to reach for eyeglasses or wear contacts on a daily basis. The best way to determine whether it is the right surgical procedure for you is to have a consultation and exam with an experienced LASIK surgeon.

Typically, you must be at least 18 years of age, have a stable eye prescription for the last year, and have healthy eyes. Patients with certain medical conditions and women who are pregnant or who are nursing may not be good candidates for this procedure.

The only way to know for certain whether you are a good candidate for this procedure or whether it is right for you is to schedule a consultation and have your eyes evaluated. During this evaluation, your eyes will be assessed and you will be presented with information to help you decide whether this is the right course of action based on your unique situation.

HOW DO I KNOW IF I'M A GOOD CANDIDATE TO HAVE LASIK?

This is one of the most frequently asked questions about LASIK. It is important for you to come in for an evaluation and consultation to determine whether you may be a good candidate for laser vision correction. While there are some general guidelines, the only way to know for certain whether this procedure may be appropriate for you is to have a consultation.

ARE ALL PATIENTS WHO WEAR CONTACTS AND EYEGLASSES GOOD CANDIDATES FOR LASIK?

Most people who wear eyeglasses are good candidates to undergo LASIK. Patients with practically every degree of nearsightedness are able to enjoy a good outcome with laser vision correction surgery. Mild to moderate degrees of nearsightedness, astigmatism, and farsightedness can be treated with LASIK. In cases of more extreme farsightedness and nearsightedness, there are other alternatives.

WHAT HAPPENS IF I MOVE MY EYE DURING THE PROCEDURE?

Thanks to the use of the latest and most advanced technology, any involuntary eye movements you might make during the procedure will not pose any threat to the procedure. The laser devices are capable of tracking both voluntary and involuntary eye movements. In fact, these lasers can track movements up to tens of thousands of times per second. They can also make any adjustments that may be necessary to put the laser back on track.

WHEN SHOULD I EXPECT MY VISION TO IMPROVE FOLLOWING MY PROCEDURE?

Most patients can expect to experience clearer vision within 24 hours of their procedure. More stabilized vision will occur over the next several weeks. In most instances, it takes a maximum of six months for the final outcomes to be apparent after the healing process has progressed.

WHAT ARE THE BENEFITS OF LASIK EYE SURGERY?

The benefits of LASIK eye surgery are being able to see clearly without having to cope with the hassles of contact lenses or glasses. This can include handling occupational tasks with more ease, participating in sports, and simply enjoying daily activities. For most patients, having LASIK performed can be a life-changing experience.

WILL I NEED TO HAVE MY EYES PATCHED?

No, it will not be necessary for you to have your eyes patched during the day. However, at night, you will be asked to wear eye patches for a few days. You will also be advised not to rub your eyes, as this can potentially create problems with the flap. In addition, you will need to follow up with your surgeon the day after your procedure to ensure your eyes are healing properly. Keep in mind that even if your eyes are not patched, you will not be able to drive yourself home following your procedure and will instead need to make arrangements to have someone drive you home as well as to your follow-up procedure.

WILL I NEED TO WEAR CONTACT LENSES OR GLASSES AFTER MY PROCEDURE?

Prior to undergoing LASIK, it is important to ensure that you have realistic expectations. Many people expect they will be able to get rid of their contact lenses or glasses completely. Instead of looking at this surgery as a way of throwing away your contacts or glasses, you should instead look at it as a way of reducing your dependence on them. It's important to remember that results do vary from one patient to another. You and your surgeon should reach an understanding on what you vision goals are prior to agreeing to surgery.

IS LASIK SAFE?

Complications in this procedure are rare. The FDA has recognized both PRK and LASIK as being quite safe and effective. Numerous safeguards have been put into place to reduce the risk of complication or error. Studies have shown that the incidence of complications such as nighttime glare or dry eyes is between 3 and 5 percent. There are no known risks of blindness associated with this procedure. Overall, the risk for complications that would threaten your sight are quite low. Even so, it is important to understand that this is a surgical procedure that does carry some risks. For this reason, it is important to do your research and select a LASIK surgeon who is well respected and experienced. When talking to prospective physicians, be sure to have a list of questions to ask.

IS LASIK PAINFUL?

Most patients report feeling no pain during their LASIK procedure. Prior to the beginning of the surgery, anesthetic drops will be used to numb your eye. You may feel a slight pressure around the eye during the procedure. If necessary, you can also be provided with a mild sedative before the procedure to help you relax.

Following your laser vision surgery, you may feel a little irritation for a few hours. After taking a short nap, most patients feel quite comfortable. You will be given prescription eye drops to promote comfort and healing following your procedure.

CAN I HAVE BOTH EYES TREATED AT THE SAME TIME?

Yes. Typically, treating both eyes at the same time is recommended.

HOW LONG WILL THE RESULTS FOR MY VISION CORRECTION SURGERY LAST?

The distance vision correction from laser vision correction is usually permanent. You should be aware that there are some age-related changes that may take place regardless of whether you have had this surgery or not.

WHAT HAPPENS DURING A LASIK EVALUATION?

During your LASIK evaluation, you should plan to be at the LASIK center for two to three hours. During this time, special tests will be used to measure as well as evaluate your eyes. You will need to stop wearing contact lenses for a period of time prior to your scheduled evaluation. Also, you should expect your eyes to be dilated during the evaluation. This is done to evaluate your refractive error along with evaluating your cornea and pupil size. You will also have a thorough discussion of what to expect with laser eye surgery and whether you are a good candidate for this procedure. In addition to meeting the surgical counselor, you should expect to have a discussion with the LASIK surgeon.

WHAT ARE THE SIDE EFFECTS OF LASIK?

The temporary side effects following laser vision correction surgery include sensitivity to light, dryness of eyes, and halos at night. Halos or glares at night typically resolve within a few weeks of having your surgery. Night vision disturbances related to imperfections in the eye prior to your surgery can be reduced or even eliminated thanks to the introduction of custom technology. Dry eyes experienced during the healing process can be treated with the use of artificial tears. It is advisable to wear sunglasses when you are outdoors after your surgery in order to reduce sensitivity to light while also protecting your eyes. As is the case with any other elective procedure, individual results may vary. There also may be additional risks related to having LASIK or PRK surgery. Such risks include undercorrection or overcorrection. With that said, the risk of complications associated with laser vision surgery is minimal.

HOW LONG DOES LASIK TAKE?

The laser treatment takes less than one minute to perform. The entire procedure usually only takes about 15 minutes per eye. Most people are quite surprised at how fast the procedure is and how good they feel after the procedure is completed.

WHEN WILL I BE ABLE TO RESUME DRIVING?

Most LASIK patients resume driving immediately after their one-day postoperative appointment.

MAY I RETURN TO WORK IMMEDIATELY?

Most patients who have LASIK are able to return to work immediately following their one-day postoperative appointment.

HOW MANY CHECKUPS WILL BE NECESSARY AFTER LASIK?

You will likely need to return for a checkup the day after your procedure and then one week later, a month later, and six months later. You should also expect to return annually after your procedure.

IF I HAVE CATARACTS, CAN LASIK FIX THEM?

It should be noted that LASIK surgery will not correct vision loss that is caused by cataracts. There are several outstanding options for persons in need of cataract surgery who want to be glasses-free.

IF I HAVE THIN CORNEAS, CAN I HAVE LASIK?

LASIK surgery is performed by reshaping the cornea with the use of an ultraprecise laser. Corneal tissue is removed as part of this process. Detailed measurements will need to be performed to make certain you have enough corneal thickness for the procedure to be performed safely. In some instances, if your corneas are too thin, you may not be a good candidate for laser vision correction surgery.

If your corneas are irregularly shaped or thin or if you have an eyeglass prescription that is very strong, you may not be a good candidate for LASIK because a significant amount of corneal thickness would need to be removed.

A symptom of dry eyes and allergies can also include chronic itchy eyes. If you have been told that you have thin corneas or if you rub your eyes often, you should discuss this with your surgeon.

Even if you are not a good candidate for LASIK because you have thin corneas, you may still be suitable for other types of procedures.

IS IT POSSIBLE TO HAVE LASIK IF I'M PREGNANT?

Most LASIK surgeons will not perform LASIK on persons who are pregnant or nursing.

CAN GLAUCOMA BE CORRECTED WITH LASIK?

Glaucoma, which often results in fields of vision loss, is often treatable with medication, laser eye surgery, or outpatient surgery. However, LASIK is not the type of laser surgery that repairs glaucoma.

CAN AMBLYOPIA OR STRABISMUS BE CORRECTED WITH LASIK?

LASIK does not correct eye muscle disorders. It is recommended to see an ophthalmologist with fellowship training in pediatric ophthalmology and strabismus.

CAN MACULAR DEGENERATION BE CORRECTED WITH LASIK?

While there are several treatments for the wet form of macular degeneration, including laser eye surgery, LASIK is not the form of laser surgery that stops progressive vision loss due to macular degeneration.

CAN ASTIGMATISM BE FIXED WITH LASIK?

LASIK can be used to correct astigmatism in most cases. The effects are usually permanent. Although it sounds somewhat frightening, astigmatism is actually quite common. It is a refractive error just like farsightedness and nearsightedness. It can be corrected with eyeglasses, contact lenses, as well as LASIK.

Astigmatism usually results from the cornea having an asymmetrical shape. The ultraprecise lasers used in LASIK can reshape the cornea so it is more symmetrical, which can help eliminate vision problems, including astigmatism. It is even possible to correct higher amounts of astigmatism with LASIK. This could increase the chances that a follow-up enhancement may be necessary to fine-tune your correction.

IS IT POSSIBLE TO IMPROVE MY READING VISION WITH LASIK?

Many people begin struggling to read small print once they reach the age of 40. This is an age-related vision problem known as presbyopia. Modern LASIK can help improve reading vision problems resulting from presbyopia.

WHAT EFFECT WILL LASIK HAVE ON MY NIGHT VISION?

Research has shown that LASIK is quite effective and safe for the correction of astigmatism, farsightedness, and nearsightedness. Many people who make the decision to have this procedure report their night vision is much sharper following LASIK than it was prior to the procedure. As part of your LASIK consultation, your physician will take detailed measurements of your eyes. During that consultation, your specific risk of halos, glares, and other side effects will be assessed and discussed with you.

IS THERE A CHANCE I WILL GO BLIND IF I HAVE LASIK?

Within the last couple of decades, millions of LASIK procedures have been performed around the world. The risk of vision-threatening complications is extremely rare. This is particularly true if you attend all follow-up visits and follow the post-op instructions provided to you. With that said, it is important to keep in mind that LASIK is still a surgical procedure. Therefore, there is some risk that complications could occur.

The complications and risks associated with this procedure are actually quite rare and can be managed. The most commonly reported complications are glare, halos, dry eyes, and visual disturbances. More severe complications, such as vision loss, may be possible but are very rare. When selecting a surgeon to perform your LASIK surgery, it's important to conduct due diligence and ask questions during your consultation to ensure you find a surgeon you feel comfortable having perform your procedure.

Your suitability for LASIK will be discussed during your preoperative consultation. This conversation will include your risk factors along with your refractive error, your age, health, and the measurements of your corneas.

WILL I BE AWAKE DURING THE PROCEDURE?

There is no need for general anesthesia because the procedure typically takes about 10 minutes to complete.

WILL IT BE NECESSARY FOR ME TO HAVE EYE EXAMS FOLLOWING LASIK?

Yes, you will need to have annual eye exams following your surgery. Along with ensuring your vision remains stable, having comprehensive eye exams on a routine basis are necessary to protect the health of your eyes. Eye exams will be required to check for any problems that could threaten your vision, including macular degeneration, glaucoma, diabetic eye disease, and cataracts. It should be noted that your risk for developing these problems does not increase by having LASIK, but the procedure also does not decrease your risk. Therefore, it's important to have routine eye exams to detect such problems early and ensure they can be treated properly.

Due to the fact that the shape and thickness of the cornea is altered by LASIK, it is also vital that you have eye exams on a routine basis to monitor the cornea's health.

If you find that you are having problems with irritated or itchy eyes, it's important to see your eye doctor to ask about available treatments. You should also make a point of wearing sunglasses to protect your eyes from harmful UV rays, which could increase your risk for developing macular degeneration or cataracts.

WHAT CAN I EXPECT IN TERMS OF THE RECOVERY TIME FOR LASIK?

You can expect your eyes to begin healing immediately following your procedure. Many people are quite surprised to discover how fast their eyes heal after LASIK. It is normal to experience some fluctuations in your vision and blurred vision for several weeks after having LASIK. This could even last for several months. You will usually be seen by your surgeon the day after your procedure to check and make sure your eyes are healing as they should. Most people are able to return to work the day after their procedure.

Regular follow-up visits will be required and are usually scheduled for about every six months to monitor your eye health and vision. Your vision should be clear and stable at the six-month checkpoint after your surgery. If you have experienced any problems with glare, halos, dry eyes, or visual disturbances, they should either be significantly reduced or gone completely by this point.

HOW OLD DO I NEED TO BE TO HAVE LASIK?

At a minimum, you should be at least 18 years old to have LASIK performed. In some instances, it may be better to wait even longer to have this procedure performed. This is because it's important for your eyes to be stable. The amount of your refractive error, whether it is astigmatism, farsightedness, or nearsightedness, needs to be stable. In most cases, myopia usually worsens during childhood. It can even continue worsening into early adulthood. You should have eye exams on an annual basis for a minimum of two years prior to having LASIK surgery. If your myopia is shown to worsen following your procedure, you may need an enhancement procedure to restore your clear vision.

HOW SOON AFTER MY SURGERY CAN I RESUME NORMAL ACTIVITIES?

The restrictions following laser surgery are quite minimal. Most patients are able to resume their normal activities the day after the procedure. The results from the procedure are usually quite fast, and many patients find they are able to see clearly within 48 hours. Over the next several months, you should experience further improvement in your vision. You will likely be advised to avoid certain activities, such as contact sports and swimming for the next several weeks.

Bathing and showering: You will be able to bathe or shower the day after your procedure, but it's important to be careful and avoid getting water or soap in your eyes for at least one week.

Exercising: You may begin exercising within a few days. Take care not to have sweat run into your eyes. You should avoid heavy lifting or other exercises that may cause you to squint or otherwise squeeze your facial muscles for about two weeks.

Swimming and hot tubs: You should wait at least two weeks.

Flying in an airplane: This is typically okay as soon as your one-day postoperative appointment is over. However, it is important that you are able to return to your surgeon's office for the next scheduled postoperative appointment.

Keep in mind that these are general guidelines and may vary based on your specific situation. Be sure to discuss it with your surgeon.

IS LASIK COVERED BY INSURANCE?

Due to the fact that LASIK is considered to be an elective procedure, it is usually not covered by insurance. With that said, you may be able to take advantage of other payment and financing options to cover the cost of your laser vision correction procedure. Also, many employers and health insurance companies offer a LASIK discount percentage.

CAN I BE PROVIDED WITH A GUARANTEE FOR MY PROCEDURE'S SUCCESS?

As is the case with any surgical procedure, there are no guarantees. There are risks associated with having any type of surgical procedure. LASIK has been performed on millions of patients with a high degree of success.

WILL ANYONE BE ABLE TO TELL THAT I'VE HAD LASIK BY LOOKING AT MY EYES?

The appearance of your eyes will not be affected by this procedure. No one will be able to tell by looking at you that you have had the procedure.

GLOSSARY OF TERMS

Ablate – To remove.

Ablation zone – The area to be removed during laser surgery.

Aberrations – Refers to distortions in waves or light rays while passing through the cornea and lens to reach the retina. Results from imperfections or irregularities along the visual pathway.

Aberrometer – A device used for creating detailed measurements of higher- and lower-order aberrations.

Accommodation – The eye's ability to change focus from distant to near objects.

Acuity – Sharpness or clearness of vision.

Age-related macular degeneration – Refers to a group of conditions that result in a loss of sharp vision. There are two types of age-related macular degeneration. They are dry and wet. This is the most common cause of decreased vision after the age of 60.

Axis – Direction of the astigmatism in degrees.

All-laser LASIK – Also referred to as bladeless LASIK, a procedure in which a laser keratome is used to create a corneal flap.

Anesthesia – Drugs used to provide numbness in specific areas of the body.

Anesthetic drops – Numbing drops placed on the eye before laser vision surgery to reduce discomfort during the surgery.

Anterior chamber angle – Refers to the junction of the iris's front surface and the cornea's back surface. This is where aqueous fluid filters from the eye.

Anterior chamber – Refers to a fluid-filled space located between the innermost corneal surface and the iris.

Aphakia – Refers to an absence of the crystalline lens.

Asthenopia – Discomfort in the eye due to use of the eyes. May include headaches and eyestrain. Could be due to a refractive error that has not been corrected.

Astigmatism – When an image is distorted on the retina resulting from irregularities in the lens or cornea.

Best-corrected visual acuity – BCVA. Refers to the best possible vision that can be achieved with corrective lenses.

Bifocals – Glasses that feature two different powers in each lens, typically for distance and near corrections.

Bilateral LASIK – When LASIK is performed on both eyes.

Bladeless LASIK – A form of LASIK in which a femtosecond laser is used to create the corneal flap. The corneal flap is then folded back so the excimer laser can provide vision correction treatment to the underlying cornea layer.

Blepharitis – Inflammation of the eyelids. May include itching, redness, and swelling.

Cataract – When the natural crystalline lens has become cloudy. This type of clouding usually occurs as part of the aging process, but may also result from inflammation, infection, or trauma.

Cataract surgery – Removing a natural lens that has become clouded and replacing it using an intraocular lens implant.

Central vision – The best vision of the eye. Helpful for discerning color and fine detail.

Cornea – The front, clear part of the eye. This is the portion of the eye responsible for bending or refracting light. The cornea offers the majority of the eye's focusing power.

Corneal flap – The first step in a LASIK surgery. Involves creating a flap within the cornea.

Crystalline lens – The natural lens in the eye that assists in delivering rays of light so they can focus on the retina.

Diabetic retinopathy – The retinal changes that occur due to diabetes mellitus.

Dilated pupil – An enlarged pupil that is caused by the dilator muscle contracting or the iris sphincter relaxing. Typically occurs in dimly lit situations or could be the result of the use of certain types of drugs, especially eye drops used in the eye doctor's office. May also result from blunt trauma.

Dilation – Widening the pupil. The eye dilates naturally to make it possible to see in lower light situations. Dilation can also be done with the use of eye drops so that the back of the eye can be examined.

Diopter – Refers to the measurement of the eye's refractive error. A negative diopter value indicates myopia while a positive diopter value indicates hyperopia.

Dry eye syndrome – When the eyes are not capable of producing enough tears to ensure the eye is kept comfortable and moist. Symptoms of this common condition may include stinging, pain, scratchiness, burning, and blurring of vision.

Endothelium – The inner layer of cells lining the interior surface of the cornea.

Epithelium – The outer layer of cells located inside the cornea. The epithelium provides protection against infection.

Excimer laser – An ultraviolet laser used to remove corneal tissue in refractive surgery.

Farsightedness – Also known as hyperopia.

FDA – The Food and Drug Administration; responsible for evaluating and approving medical devices.

Femtosecond laser – A laser that features a short pulse time. Used for creating flaps in bladeless LASIK procedures as well as in laser-assisted cataract procedures.

Flexible spending account – A health savings account provided by employers, which allows employees to take advantage of tax advantages while setting aside money for qualified expenditures. LASIK is eligible for such expenditures.

Floaters – Particles that float in the vitreous. Occurs as a result of aging or with inflammation.

Glare – Scatter that occurs from bright light. Causes vision to decrease.

Glaucoma – A condition that often results in some vision loss.

Halos – Rings that occur around lights as a result of optical imperfections located in the front of the eye.

Haze – Clouding that occurs in the cornea, causing vision to appear like looking through fog or smoke.

Health savings account – An account created for individuals who have a high deductible health plan. With this plan, it's possible to save for medical expenses that would not be covered by a high-deductible health plan. Contributions may be made by individuals and/or their employer. Yearly limits do apply. This type of plan offers certain tax advantages.

Hyperopia – The inability to see near objects as well as distant objects.

Inflammation – How the body responds to infection, trauma, or the presence of a foreign substance. May result in heat, pain, swelling, or redness.

Intraocular – Within the eye.

Intraocular pressure – The amount of pressure within the eye can be measured based on the amount of aqueous fluid that is created and then drained inside the eye. Increased intraocular pressure can place pressure on the optic nerve. This can result in significant vision problems. A tonometer is used to measure intraocular pressure.

IOL – Also known as intraocular lens. This is an artificial lens that replaces the eye's natural crystalline lens, usually when the natural lens becomes cloudy due to a cataract. Once the natural lens is removed and replaced with an IOL, the eye is able to properly focus light onto the retina.

Iris – The colored ring located behind the cornea and in front of the lens.

Irregular astigmatism – Irregular or distorted curvature of the cornea. Causes blurry vision.

Keratectomy – Surgically removing corneal tissue.

Keratotomy – Making a surgical cut or incision in the cornea.

Keratitis – Corneal inflammation.

Keratoconus – An irregularly or cone-shaped corneal surface that results in distorted, blurred images.

Keratomileusis – Reshaping the cornea.

Laser – An instrument used to produce a beam of light used for vaporizing tissue.

Laser keratome – A laser used specifically for creating corneal flaps.

LASIK – Laser assisted in situ keratomileusis. The creation of a flap in the cornea with the use of a microkeratome and laser for the purpose of reshaping the cornea.

Lens – The part of the eye responsible for providing focusing power. The lens has the ability to change shapes, which makes it possible for the eye to focus at varying distances.

Lid speculum –An instrument used to hold the eyelids apart and prevent the patient from blinking during the procedure.

Lower-order aberrations – Also known as refractive errors, including astigmatism, hyperopia, and myopia.

Microkeratome – A surgical device that is positioned on the eye using a vacuum ring. Used to cut into the cornea at predetermined depths. Older microkeratomes use a blade.

Monofocal lens – An intraocular lens implant that makes it possible to enjoy clear vision at a specific distance.

Monovision – Deliberately treating one eye for near vision and the other eye for distance vision.

Multifocal lens – An intraocular lens implant that works similarly to a trifocal or bifocal lens in eyeglasses. Provides clear vision at multiple distances.

Myopia – An inability to view distant objects as clearly as near objects.

Nearsightedness – Also known as myopia.

Ophthalmologist – A physician who attended medical or osteopathic school and specializes in medical and surgical diagnosis and treatment of eye diseases and vision disorders.

Optician – Someone who specializes in making and fitting eyeglasses and dispensing contact lenses.

Optical zone – The center of the cornea. This is where laser photoablation occurs. The size of the optical zone may range from 5 to 9 mm based on the type of laser that is used.

Optometrist – A physician who attended optometry school and who diagnoses, manages, and treats eye diseases and vision disorders.

Overcorrection – A complication of refractive surgery in which there is more correction performed than necessary.

Photobia – An abnormal sensitivity to light. Sometimes linked with excessive tearing. Usually due to the cornea or iris being inflamed.

Ptosis – Drooping of the upper eyelid. Could be due to a weakness of the cranial nerve or may be congenital.

Postoperative – The healing period following a LASIK procedure. During this time, it's important for patients to adhere to certain requirements.

PRK – Also known as photorefractive keratectomy. Removal of the epithelium or the surface layer of the cornea. The procedure is performed by scraping the surface layer gently using a computer-controlled excimer laser.

Presbyopia – When the eye is not able to maintain a clear image as objects move nearer. This is an age-related condition that results from reduced elasticity in the lens.

Pupil – A hole located in the center of the iris. In response to changes in lighting, the pupil changes in size. For instance, the pupil becomes larger in low-light settings and becomes smaller in brighter lighting situations.

Radial keratotomy – Also known as RK. This surgical procedure uses radial cuts to flatten the cornea and correct myopia.

Refraction – A test used for determining the eye's refractive power. This term also refers to the light bending as it passes from medium to medium.

Refractive errors – Imperfections in the eye's focusing power. Includes hyperopia, presbyopia, astigmatism, and myopia.

Refractive power – The ability of the eye to bend light.

Retina – A layer of tissue lining the interior wall of the eye. In many ways, the retina is similar to film in a camera that is used for capturing images. Those images are then transformed into electrical signals and transmitted to the brain.

Retinal detachment – Separation of the retina from the underlying epithelium.

Sclera – The white outer coating of the eyeball. Offers protection to the eyeball.

Snellen visual acuity chart – The most common chart used for measuring vision.

Striae – Also known as folds, these are wrinkles that occur in the corneal flap after a LASIK procedure. This complication can be corrected by irrigating or lifting under the flap and then repositioning the flap.

Stroma – The thick, middle layer of tissue located inside the cornea.

Topography – Refers to a topographical map of the eye's surface that is created in order to assess the cornea's shape. Topography is used during an evaluation to determine whether the eye is stable enough to undergo surgery.

Toric lens – An intraocular lens implant or contact lens used to correct astigmatism.

Undercorrection – A complication that may occur in refractive surgery. Occurs when not enough correction is provided.

Visual acuity – Clear vision; the ability to distinguish shapes and details.

Vitreous humor – The transparent gel that is positioned behind the lens and located in front of the retina.

Wavefront – Measures the total amount of refractive error in the eye.

CONCLUSION

Making the decision to have LASIK is an important one that can have a profound impact on your life. If you have relied on the use of eyeglasses or contact lenses, then you know how frustrating it can be. In many cases, wearing contact lenses or glasses can limit or interfere with your daily activities. While there are no guarantees that having LASIK will allow you to eliminate your glasses or contact lenses, this procedure could certainly help to reduce your reliance on them.

When considering having LASIK, as is the case with any surgical procedure, it's important to make sure you are well informed about the procedure, how it is performed, and the potential risks associated with that procedure. It's also imperative that you take the time to find a surgeon with the right amount of experience and whom you feel comfortable having perform your procedure.

There is absolutely no need to continue living with the hassles of eyeglasses or contact lenses when there are options available to reduce or even eliminate your reliance on them. Not everyone is a good candidate for laser vision correction, but the only way to find out whether you could be a good candidate for LASIK is to schedule an appointment and have your eyes evaluated. Even if you are not a good candidate for LASIK, there could be alternate procedures that could help to improve your vision.

Overall, the advantages of LASIK are quite numerous. Compared to the long-term costs associated with wearing glasses or contact lenses for the rest of your life, LASIK can also be affordable. A variety of other financing options may also be available to help defray the cost of laser vision correction surgery.

If you have been considering having LASIK, there has never been a better time.

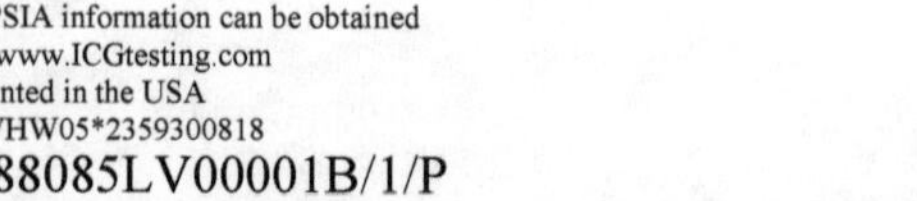

CPSIA information can be obtained
at www.ICGtesting.com
Printed in the USA
LVHW05*2359300818
588085LV00001B/1/P